Great Books

by

Pulitzer and Nobel Prize Nominee

E. S. Abramson

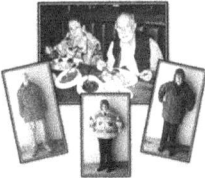

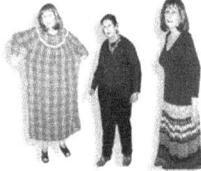

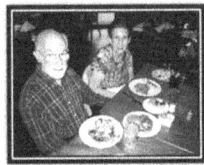

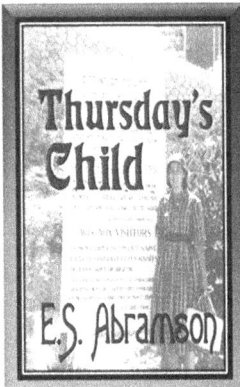

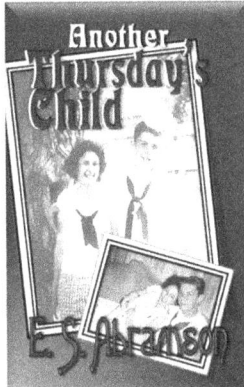

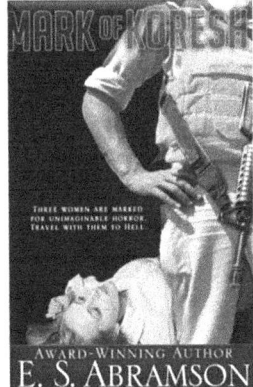

Visit Red Carpet Press
online at
www.Red-Carpet-Press.com

Keep up on our latest new
releases from your favorite
authors, as well as author
appearances, news, blogs,
chats, special offers and
more.

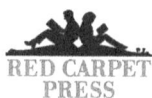

RED CARPET
PRESS

"Rolling Out the 'Read' Carpet, One Fantastic Book at a Time.™"

WE WENT FROM
FAT TO FABULOUS TOGETHER:
A DIET GUIDE FOR RESTAURANT LOVERS
E. S. Abramson

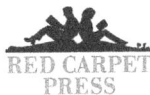

RED CARPET
PRESS

"Rolling Out the 'Read' Carpet, One Fantastic Book at a Time.™"

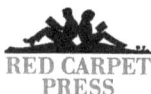

RED CARPET
PRESS
Hazelwood, MO

"Rolling Out the 'Read' Carpet, One Fantastic Book at a Time.™"

THE NATIONAL LEAGUE OF AMERICAN PEN WOMEN • PEN ARTS BUILDING • 1300 17TH STREET, nw • WASHINGTON, dc 20036-1973 • TELEPHONE (202) 785-1997

Fax: 1-202-452-6868   e-mail: NLAPW1@juno.com

CONDUCTING AND PROMOTING PROFESSIONAL WORK IN ART • LETTERS • MUSIC SINCE 1897

The Pulitzer Prize Office
Columbia University
709 Pulitzer Hall
2950 Broadway, New
York, New York 10027

Dear Pulitzer Prize Administrator:

I would like to nominate Elaine Abramson's *From Fat to Fabulous: A Diet Guide for Restaurant Lovers* for this year's Pulitzer Prize.

With the World Health Organization reporting that 13% of all Americans are overweight or are obese and America is number one with the most overweight or obese people in the world, I think a book that gives people the incentive and the tools to help them lose weight is a worthy candidate for this award.

Thank you for considering Ms. Abramson's book.

Thelma H. Urich

Thelma H. Urich
President of the St. Louis Branch of the National League of American Pen Women
Past President of the Missouri State Association of NLAPW
Former National New Letters Chairman of NLAPW

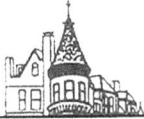

The National League of American Pen Women (NLAPW), founded in 1897, is the oldest and one of the most prestigious organizations in the world for women in art, letters, and music. NLAPW's headquarters is in the historic Robert Todd Lincoln house in Washington, D.C.

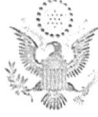

On June 16, 2014, "Dr. Mehmet Oz appeared before the Senate's consumer protection panel and was scolded by Chairman Claire McCaskill for claims he made about weight-loss aids on his TV show, 'The Dr. Oz Show.'" – Associated Press.

On August 8, 2014 Senator Claire McCaskill endorsed *FROM FAT TO FABULOUS: A DIET GUIDE FOR RESTAURANT LOVERS*.

EAT, <u>DRINK</u> AND BE **_MERRY_**, and have **F<u>U</u>N** on the *FROM FAT TO FABULOUS*™ restaurant lovers' diet.

A big thank you to my fantastic husband Stan Abramson for all the time he spent editing, living with, and loving me as I went *FROM FAT TO FABULOUS*™. He had so much faith in my restaurant lover's diet that he went *FROM FAT TO FABULOUS*™ along with me.

I would also like to thank Thelma H. Urich, a great friend and mentor, for her belief in me and my restaurant lover's diet.

CONTENTS

CONTENTS

CONTENTS

CONTENTS

CONTENTS

APPEARANCES, ARTICLES, AND ENDORSEMENTS

"I WOULD LIKE TO NOMINATE Elaine Abramson's *From Fat to Fabulous: A Diet Guide for Restaurant Lovers* series for this year's **Pulitzer Prize**. I think a book that gives people the incentive and the tools to help them lose weight is a worthy candidate for this award." Thelma H. Urich, President of the St. Louis Branch of the National League of American Pen Women (NLAPW), Past President of the Missouri State Association of NLAPW, and Former National New Letters Chairman of NLAPW.

U.S. Senator Claire McCaskill endorsed *From Fat to Fabulous: A Diet Guide for Restaurant Lovers* saying, "Creating this book required a considerable amount of hard work and dedication. You should be proud of your accomplishment."

Missouri Governor Jay Nixon endorsed *From Fat to Fabulous: A Diet Guide for Restaurant Lovers,* the **ONLY FUN** and **ENJOYABLE DIET.** "It is my honor to congratulate you on the completion of your book *From Fat to Fabulous: A Diet Guide for Restaurant Lovers.* Your book is a great resource for those who enjoy dining out, while still maintaining a healthy lifestyle."

Albuquerque Mayor Richard Berry also endorsed *From Fat to Fabulous: A Diet Guide for Restaurant Lovers.* "Your accomplishment of losing 85 pounds and 10 dress sizes while eating only restaurant meals is truly remarkable. Enjoying dining out is not something that the residence of the city should have to give up to maintain a healthy lifestyle. Your book will be very beneficial in educating the residents of the city on how to pick healthy, well-balanced and delicious meals while at the same time being able to enjoy socializing at their favorite dining establishments."

APPEARANCES

KASEY JOYCE, MULTIMEDIA TELEVISION JOURNALIST, reviewed *From Fat to Fabulous: A Diet Guide for Restaurant Lovers* on KSDK-TV (NBC-TV). Also posted the interview on KSDK.com. http://www.ksdk.com/news/article/290001/3/Local-woman-dropped-50-pounds-on-restaurant-diet.

Featured Health News Video on KSDK.com. **"Local woman dropped 50 pounds on restaurant diet."** http://www.ksdk.com/video/default.aspx?bctid=1319110982001&odyssey=mod|newswell|text|FRONTPAGE|featured.

From Fat to Fabulous: A Diet Guide for Restaurant Lovers was on KDNL-TV (ABC-TV).

Featured Health News Video on KSDK.com. "Local woman dropped 50 pounds on restaurant diet."

From Fat to Fabulous: A Diet Guide for Restaurant Lovers was featured on KOB-TV (NBC) Good Morning New Mexico.

FoodTalkSTL on KFNS-AM radio 590 – Elaine Abramson, a woman who lost 85 pounds by *only eating restaurant food!*

Cape Girardeau Storytelling Festival – *From Fat to Fabulous: A Diet Guide for Restaurant Lovers.*

ARTICLES

R IVERFRONT TIMES BLOG – BOOKS – "LOCAL **Author <u>Drops 10 Dress Sizes</u> on 'Restaurant Diet'.**

http://blogs.riverfronttimes.com/gutcheck/2011/12/elaine_abramsonr estaurant_diet.php. "By eating only restaurant meals, E. S. Abramson lost 85 pounds and went from a size 22 to a size 12. She believes she has stumbled onto the world's greatest diet and that if everyone followed her example, we'd all be thinner and healthier."

The KSDK-TV, KDNL-TV, and the Riverfront Times Blog can also be found on www.ElaineAbramson.com.

Featured in the St. Louis Post-Dispatch – Health News – **"Woman leaves own kitchen to shape up….. DIETITIANS HAIL PLAN"**: http://www.stltoday.com/lifestyles/health-med-fit/fitness/woman-leaves-own-kitchen-to-shape-up/article_78700114-f099-5153-b7c0-1ac5ca1a6afe.html#ixzz1sQoR3WbD

St. Louis Post-Dispatch – Elaine Abramson – http://www.stltoday.com/lifestyles/health-med-fit/fitness/elaine-abramson/article_e5dafb01-ca76-582a-837f-6102fff72d83.html#ixzz1sVBCrtWX

Huffpost Blog http://www.huffingtonpost.com/social/Elaine_Abramson/weight-loss-success-yvette-nathan-jones_n_1193965_131163670.html

FoodTalkSTL on KFNS-AM radio 590 – Elaine Abramson, a woman who lost 85 pounds by *only eating restaurant food!*

PBS Blog – http://www.pbs.org/newshour/bb/health/jan-june12/obesity_05-08.html

HBO Blog – http://www.mediaowners.com/company/hbo.html

Newsweek Blog –
http://www.thedailybeast.com/newsweek/2012/05/06/why-the-campaign-to-stop-america-s-obesity-crisis-keeps-failing.html

Cape Girardeau Storytelling Festival. Also taped for PBS Cape Girardeau.

ENDORSEMENTS

HEALTH ENDORSEMENTS

"ELAINE IS OUR DIET DIVA! She is inspirational." – *Cathy Cummings, Nurse, St. Louis Orthopedic Institute.*

"**What great work**," said *Connie Diekman, director of university nutrition at Washington University.* "She assessed her lifestyle, recognized the need for change and took action."

Amy Moore, dietetics and nutrition instructor at St. Louis University, said "Abramson seems to have **mastered making good choices**."

"After seeing Elaine's before and after pictures, I was really impressed with the results that were achieved by this diet. Sounds like a lot of fun to go out and enjoy great restaurant meals and lose weight in the process." – *Dr. Srdjan Ilic.*

RESTAURANT ENDORSEMENTS

"ELAINE'S PROVEN DIET OBVIOUSLY WORKS... Elaine looks fabulous. Amici's Restaurant staff and culinary team have been honored to help Elaine with her proven results." – *Amici's Restaurant proprietors Dave Pullam and Jim McInroy.*

"We believe that Elaine has enjoyed our food because everything is made from scratch. Our food has no preservatives and no saturated fats that you get from packaged foods. We see Elaine choose from our menu very wisely. We are happy to see that Elaine has had great success with dieting while supporting local restaurants. Thanks," – *David Miller and Tony Dahl, Partners of Dave and Tony's Premium Burger Joint.*

OTHER ENDORSEMENTS

"WITH SO MANY CHALLENGES TO our health and happiness around every corner—and on every plate—it's never been more important to be armed with knowledge and options. Elaine's story and plan will inform, amuse, and possibly even save your life." – *Tom Hall, Graphic Designer & Lifestyle Enthusiast.*

"We have known Elaine for years and she looks and feels better than ever. Kudos to Elaine and a plan that makes you feel that way." – *Walter Alston, Engineer and Pam Stiehr, Grill Chef.*

"You look fabulous!" – *Jackie D. Sclair, Insurance Agent.*

"Wow! Elaine, where did you leave your Siamese twin?" – *Chris Fulton, Senior Engineer.*

"Elaine practices what she preaches in *From Fat to Fabulous.* Looking great!" – *Thelma Urich, former National New Letters Chair for the National League of American Pen Women (NLAPW), past President of the Missouri State Association of NLAPW, president of the St. Louis branch of NLAPW.*

"The best problem solver is someone who has overcome the problem. Elaine is an overcomer who managed to reduce her size from a 22 to a svelte 12. Her practical plan is easy to follow – - but most of all it works. Bravo!" – *Robin Theiss, St. Louis Writer, Bookseller, and Business Consultant.*

"It's been a joy to watch Elaine's success story evolve. She grew from a thin, frail child to a hefty woman wearing a size 22 to a size 12 curvaceous women after losing fifty pounds in one year. With an incentive to succeed, she preserved through many popular diets only to create her own restaurant diet regimen. She has set a good example for all of her friends." – *Jeannine Dahlberg, Author.*

"You are SO inspirational, Elaine!" – *Barbara Chartier, Screenwriter.*

"So many weight loss programs rely on time-consuming meal preparation, which makes them hard for an on-the-go person to follow. Others rely on bland fare that sucks all the pleasure from eating. Elaine Abramson's Restaurant Lover's Guide offers a healthy, effective alternative for those of us who eat most of our meals between appointments." – *Jaden Terrell, Author and Executive Director of Killer Nashville Conference.*

"I am amazed at the transformation of Elaine from an attractive heavy set woman to a much slimmer lady with a beautiful figure. I think Elaine's restaurant diet is fantastic, and I plan to follow her approach to losing weight." – *Adrienne Rosen, fine artist and teacher.*

"Most people have found that eating in restaurants frequently will increase their waistlines. Elaine has found a creative way to reverse this. Elaine looks younger since she went on her diet. We should all want to have this information. Way to use your creativity!" – *Betty Shew, Artist.*

"You look amazing!" – *Maggie McCarthy, Watercolorist.*

"Thank you for sharing your story with me during lunch. It is such a delight to meet interesting people who have overcome huge obstacles in life. You are an inspiration! I look at this as "God stepping in to help you and then using you to inspire others and help others with emotional or physical conditions which keep them from experiencing joy in their lives." – *Ruth Galayda*

I've seen Elaine's restaurant diet in action – it's easy once you know what to do. And she looks great!" – *New York Times bestselling author Angie Fox.*

"Your diet gives hope and shows that others can do it, too." – *Ellie Searl, formatter of each edition of* FROM FAT TO FABULOUS: A DIET GUIDE FOR RESTAURANT LOVERS

FROM FAT TO FABULOUS: A DIET GUIDE FOR RESTAURANT LOVERS is a great resource if you love to eat out (and who doesn't?) but need to know how to eat smart. Elaine Abramson has scored with this one! – *Bill Hopkins, retired judge and author of the Judge Rosswell Carew Mystery series.*

"Another edition! Yeah! Your book has struck a chord!" – *Pam DeVoe, anthropologist and author.*

"Elaine Abramson proves you can lose weight and still eat out. She's a walking testament to smart eating by having the courage to ask for the right kind of food. FROM FAT TO FABULOUS: A DIET GUIDE FOR RESTAURANT LOVERS tells how she did it, so you can too! I highly recommend it." – *Sharon Woods Hopkins, mortgage banker and author of the Rhetta McCarter Mystery series.*

"I enjoyed the book. I am going to keep it in the car. Then when we go to different restaurants I can peek at the book and see what exchanges you made to make the meal a good one for us who are watching or trying to lose weight. Thanks again." – *Ruth Galayda.*

I WAS A FOODAHOLIC

JUST LIKE AN ALCOHOLIC CRAVES alcohol and drug addicts crave drugs, I crave food. Lots of food, especially food that put large amounts of excess weight on me. But unlike an alcoholic or a drug addict whose bodies do not need those harmful substances to survive, our bodies cannot exist and remain healthy without a sufficient amount of food and water. I had to recognize I had a problem that no one else could cure for me. I had to do it myself.

For over forty years I tried one diet after another, from the celebrity diets to the clubs diets, to elimination diets, to fad diets, to the diets my doctors gave me. None of them worked for me. Why is the *From Fat to Fabulous™* restaurant lovers' diet the only one I have ever succeeded on? Because it is **FUN** and **ENJOYABLE.**

There are no operations, no pills, and no high impact aerobics. And there is no mess, no fuss, no work, and no measuring or counting calories, carbs, or trans fats. The only thing I had to do was choose a restaurant from the listing in one of the *FROM FAT TO FABULOUS: A DIET GUIDE FOR RESTAURANT LOVERS* dining guides, order from the restaurant menu, and **ENJOY** my meal.

FROM FAT TO FABULOUS™

W AHOO! I AM THE LUCKIEST WOMAN ALIVE! At my
last annual exam my doctor said my tests indicated that my
body is ten years younger than it had been the previous year. She
credited my better health and tremendous weight loss to my restaurant
lovers' diet.

Double WAHOO! I have not set foot in my kitchen in over six
years to cook a meal. And by the grace of God I will never cook
another meal. The only time my kitchen is graced with my presence
is when I defrost my restaurant leftovers, microwave them, and sit
down to eat.

With the odds stacked against me, on the only **FUN** way to lose
weight I lost 100 pounds. I have a sluggish thyroid, do not have a
spleen, and take medicine that causes weight gain, had a slipped disk,
and have very bad knees making any form of exercise extremely
difficult.

The questions people ask most frequently about my diet are: 1)
"Won't you get fat eating in restaurants?" Answer: not if you eat the
right foods. In *FROM FAT TO FABULOUS* and *WE WENT FROM FAT TO
FABULOUS* I told readers that I had gone from a size 22 to a size 12 by
eating only in restaurants. Today I wear a size 8. 2) "Is it expensive
to eat out?" My husband is a computer programmer and I am an
author. We are middle class Americans. We eat out Friday night,
Saturday and Sunday lunch and dinner, and on special occasions. I
clip coupons out of magazines and newspapers, print them off the
Internet, and use them at restaurant chains and local independent
establishments. Our favorite coupons are the buy-one-lunch-or-dinner
and get-one-of-equal-value-free type. Second to that were the thirty,

twenty-five, and ten-dollar-off- your-total-bill coupons. We do not buy entertainment or dining books because they never seem to have the restaurants we want to eat at.

One of the most overlooked restaurant bargains is the Early Bird special. It has become more and more popular at restaurants frequented by working people. DinnerBroker.com lists numerous restaurants that will take 30% off the bill if you eat there before 6 p.m. Some restaurants will also extend this discount throughout the evening. You make reservations on the restaurant's website, and the discount is automatically applied to your bill. And 5pm.co.uk offers off-peak-time restaurant discounts up to 50% in the United Kingdom.

My husband and I come home with so many take-out boxes that our refrigerator and freezer are always full.

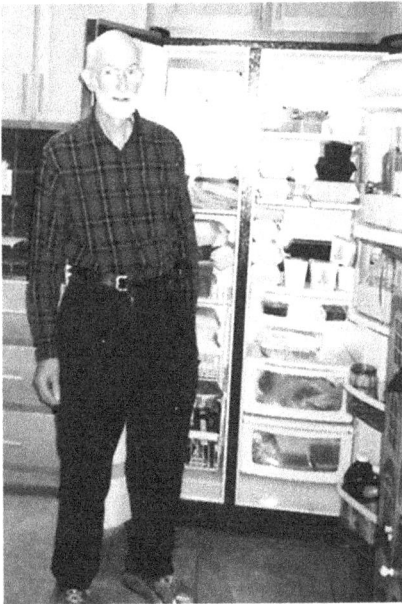

*Our refrigerator and freezer are always stocked
with restaurant food leftovers.*

By using restaurant offers and coupons and by eliminating the fat from meat that must be disposed of, oil I dumped out after sautéing meat and vegetables, peelings I threw in the garbage, meat and vegetable shrinkage during cooking, cost of using the stove and oven, cost of detergent and running the dishwasher, and all the other things I did to prepare a meal and clean up afterwards, there was only a slight difference in our food bills between what we spent in grocery stores and what we spent in restaurants. Best of all, with all these leftovers we have the convenience of not having to prepare a meal and the fun of choosing a different meal every time we eat.

I grew up in Cleveland, Ohio, a rust-belt city, a reference to the steel mills closing and the tremendous loss of jobs. Between 1929, the Depression Era, and 1945, when World War II and rationing ended, food was scarce. With an abundance of food suddenly available, mothers believed that the only healthy child was a well-fed child. You ate when you were happy. You ate when you were sad. There was never an occasion that did not include food. Clean Plate clubs with toy treasure chests sat in front of most restaurant cash registers. It was an era when Americans celebrated world peace and plenty of food on the table. No one thought about the long-term effects of being overweight.

By the time I was in my mid-sixties I had so much pain in my

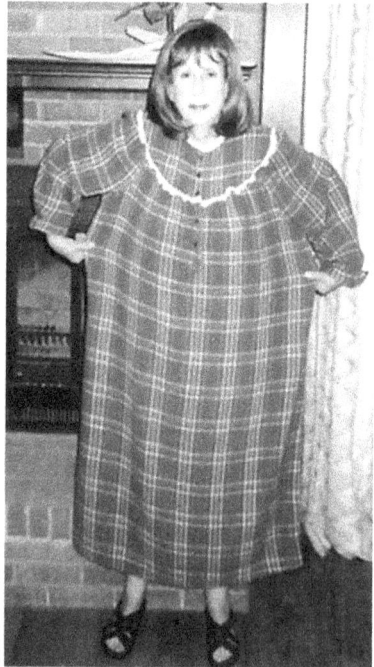

The dress I wore before I began my restaurant lover's diet

knees and ankles I could barely stand or walk. The life I knew and loved had come to a screeching halt. It was either do something about it or give up everything I wanted to do.

I believe that diets that are not fun and enjoyable are doomed to failure. If you work hard enough on the calorie-counting heavy-exercise diets, you will lose weight, but if you do not continue this regime indefinitely, like a boomerang the weight will return. You will pack on the pounds again and in some cases weigh more than you did before you began the diet.

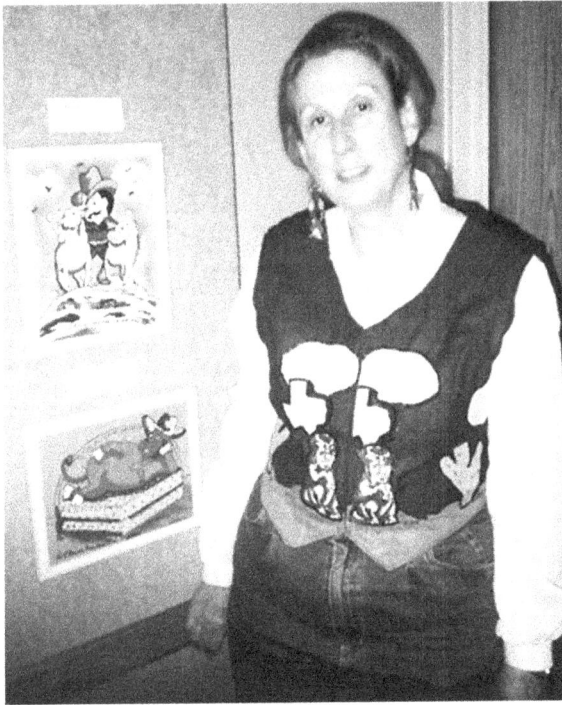

Dallas branch of the National League of American Pen Women's juried art show

What I am about to say is <u>not</u> to be taken as medical advice. It is simply to tell you how eating certain foods at certain times of the day affected me. A couple years ago I was diagnosed with fibromyalgia. I could not sleep at night because it caused tingling, severe pain, and burning. I twisted and turned in bed trying to find a way to end my torment. My podiatrist gave me cortisone shots. They did not give me any relief. He then prescribed Lyrica. Lyrica gave me some relief but caused another problem. In fourteen days I gained fourteen pounds. I figured that if I stayed on Lyrica for one year, I would have gained three hundred sixty-five pounds. The fear that all that weight gain would put so much stress on my knees that I would never walk again made me decide to stop taking Lyrica. This was followed by my podiatrist and primary care doctor prescribing other drugs and creams. They failed to give me any relief. I love dark chocolate. I ate it every day after dinner. One day I ate it after lunch instead of after dinner. That night the fibromyalgia seemed to be less severe, so for the next week I experimented. I ate the chocolate after lunch instead of after dinner. Since changing the time of day that I eat the chocolate, I rarely have a problem from fibromyalgia. I concluded that since it is important to take certain medications at certain times of the day, it may also be a good idea to eat certain foods at certain times of the day.

Because I am always on the lookout for ways to improve my diet and my health, I have become an avid magazine reader. I also watch television and internet health, diet, restaurant, and cooking shows. I also study the commercials. In this age of fast-foods, prepared foods, fast-food restaurants, and high pressure marketing I have to know which foods will make my diet work, so I check out all the information available. I want to be an informed dieter, one who will improve her health and slim down at the same time. So that you too may be an informed dieter, I have included my research.

Kitchen Daily said "the queen of England owns a McDonald's. Back in the '60s, Queen Elizabeth decided to diversify her royal portfolio and get into the restaurant franchise game, and purchased a McDonald's in Michigan." Do the Royals eat there? Probably not. Most sources claim that the entire health-conscious Royal Family is vegetarian.

AOL's article "Diet Food Backlash....Dieters move past calories" stated that "Obsessing over calories alone has left dieters with an empty feeling." And "'Low-calorie' foods make people feel deprived. Now, people want to lose weight while still feeling satisfied. And they want to do it without foods they consider processed.... dieters are sick of foods that provide only fleeting satisfaction and seem to make them hungrier. The new thinking is that eating foods with more protein or fat will make dieters less likely to binge later, even if they're higher in calories." The article went on to say that people are looking for nutritional benefits, not just reduced calories. Processed food producers such as cereal makers, soda bottlers, and prepared meal packagers claim they are adding more nutrition while subtracting calories from their products. Would they add more nutritional value to their products if their sales weren't down? I doubt it. Because additives are needed to make processed foods taste better and preservatives are used to give them longer shelf life, my husband and I do not eat prepared foods. Everything we eat must be prepared fresh and must not contain fillers, additives, or preservatives.

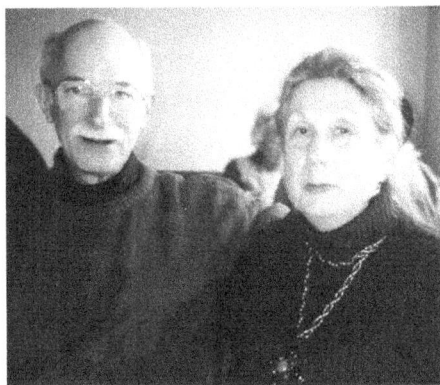

Boeing Dining Club

In *Arthritis* magazine Jennifer said, "I lost 15 pounds. That's 60 pounds of pressure off my knees." No wonder I could not walk and was in so much pain I could not stand up without crying before I started my restaurant lovers' diet. If the loss of 15 pounds took 60 pounds of pressure off Jennifer's knees, then my 85 pound loss removed 340 pounds of pressure off my knees.

Parkcrest Orthopedics advice in *St. Louis Magazine* said, "Your weight has a significant impact on your knees. Americans take an average of 4,000 steps per day on each leg. With every step, your knee supports 3.5 times your body weight. This means that if you're even just 10 pounds overweight, your knees are supporting an extra 70 pounds every day—a staggering figure that can equate to joint damage in the future." If nothing else, their figures are scary enough to discourage me from regaining any of the weight I lost.

Constantly changing restaurant menus are examples of diets that don't work. One restaurant chain switched from a celebrity doctor's diet to a low-calorie menu to a diet club diet and finally to a low-calorie diet endorsed by a diet club. I don't want to go out for a good time and have to count calories, carbs, portion sizes, or eat prepackaged or frozen dinners sized to specific diet requirements. Restaurants would not have to switch from diet to diet if they prepared meals that tasted good and helped you slim down while being fun and enjoyable at the same time.

Men's Health Magazine's "Stupid Diets...that work!" claimed Jared [the Subway guy] switched from eating junk food to eating subs with smaller portions of low-fat or fat-free condiments such as mayonnaise." He combined two vegetarian subs a day with a lot of walking. I don't know about anyone else, but I never eat low-fat or fat-free condiments. To me they are tasteless. I do not check portion size before I order. I eat until I feel full. Because I am anemic and I do not have a spleen, his vegetarian diet would never work for me. I need the iron in meat. In January 2010, *People* magazine reported that "Fogel had gained weight but was planning to restart his weight-loss program to stop the backslide and slim up."

A 2014 Today Show headline read, "Kirstie Alley joins Jenny Craig to lose weight—again." The actress, who lost her original Jenny Craig weight loss diet battle, is trying the Jenny Craig diet for the second time. She said, "I have to be more disciplined." Alley was their celebrity spokesperson for three years. Marie Osmond, speaking for Nutrisystem, admits that she has failed to succeed on her diets numerous times. Fergie, Sarah the Duchess of York, failed on the Weight Watchers diet and had to begin dieting all over again. All of these women claim to have put on fifty pounds or more after they went off those diets. Today Show nutritionist Joy Bauer has people restrict their calories, substitute low fat or low calorie foods for the foods they previously ate, and do strenuous exercises. These things never worked for me. The reason my restaurant lover's diet works for me is because, unlike the examples above, I have a diet where I did not have to be extremely disciplined, do not have to do strenuous exercises, and do not have to give up eating the foods I love. I have a diet that is **FUN** and **ENJOYABLE**, one I **ENJOY** so much that it is easy to stick to it.

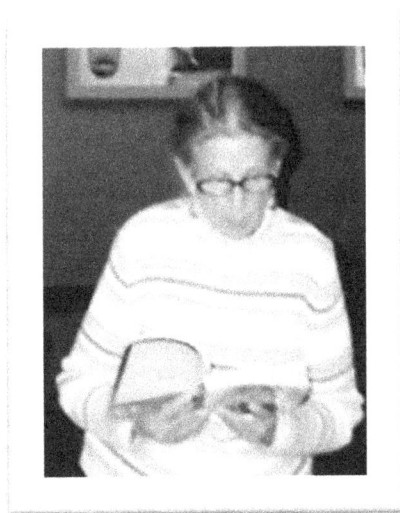

*Photo courtesy Sandy Bazinet. Writer to
Writer workshop and reading.*

Television is a great educator. The food and diet ads are especially informative. Every food producer tells you how good for you his product is because it has only a limited number of calories. Restaurant ads now brag about their low-calorie menus. I don't want to count calories. Boar's Head's meats booklet lists the calories, total fat, cholesterol, sodium and protein in their products. I would get a headache trying to keep track of all those numbers. If I loved numbers, I would have become an accountant. I just want to sit down, not have to worry about figuring out how many calories I am eating, and enjoy a meal.

What never ceases to amaze me is how confusing television messages are. Talk shows, news segments, and cooking programs present low-calorie, low-fat, and low cholesterol segments followed by ads for foods so fattening they will blow any diet out of the water. Nutritionists and doctors relate information on foods you should avoid in order to maintain your weight and health. It is followed by celebrity chefs telling you how to make cholesterol and artery clogging snacks to eat while watching TV. Before each holiday and swimsuit season, skinny nutritionists recommend eating fruits and vegetables. A celebrity follows giving you his or her favorite rich dessert recipe. Is the celebrity fat? Of course not. If he or she were fat, you would think twice about making that tempting dessert. The celebrity and the program's host will take a bite of the fattening food, "ooh" and "ahh" over it, and tell you how delicious it is. After that one bite you never see the celebrity or the program's host finish the food.

During the Sochi Olympics celebrity chef Giada De Laurentis made treats to eat while watching the games. She made spicy citrus buttered popcorn with vodka and crispy salami. Skier Lindsey Vonn gave her recipe for banana bread. The cooking segment ended with chocolate cupcake recipes and a comment about how low in calories the cupcakes were. No one mentioned the huge amounts of sugar in these treats or the nitrates and other unhealthy additives in the crispy salami.

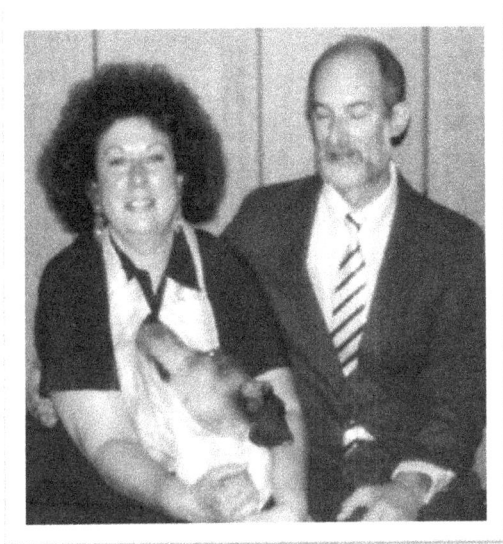

In the mid-1950's my father discovered packaged cake mixes. All he had to do was grease and flour a pan, add eggs and water, and throw it in the oven. Most of the time his cakes came out lopsided. All of my friend's mothers piled rich gooey frosting on their cakes. When I asked my father if the cakes being lopsided were the reason he did not frost them, he replied that the cakes contained so much sugar he did not need to frost them. As a teenager I thought his reasoning was ridiculous. I never saw him add any sugar to the mix, so where was all the sugar he was talking about? After I had been on my restaurant lover's diet for a couple of months, I understood what he was talking about. I could taste the sugar in the cake. It left a sweet taste in my mouth. That's when I began to realize that cake, bread, and pasta all have natural sugar in them.

Many people confuse natural sugar with the refined sugar put in coffee, tea, and other sweet beverages and cake frosting, pies, and ice cream. Natural sugar can be found in syrup and fruits and vegetables.

High carbohydrate foods like bread, pasta, potatoes, and rice also contain natural sugars and starches. They supply energy to the body, but unfortunately that energy is short lived.

As an artist, the ads I find most interesting are the ones that tell you all the ways you can dress up breakfast foods. Cereals are shown with funny faces made out of strawberries, blueberries, and other fruits. Cereal producers do this to disguise the fact that cereal is the most fattening part of your breakfast. I love the ads that say you will lose six pounds in a week if you eat their products. They never say what happens after the week is up. If it were my body, the weight would return the following week if I continued to eat the cereal.

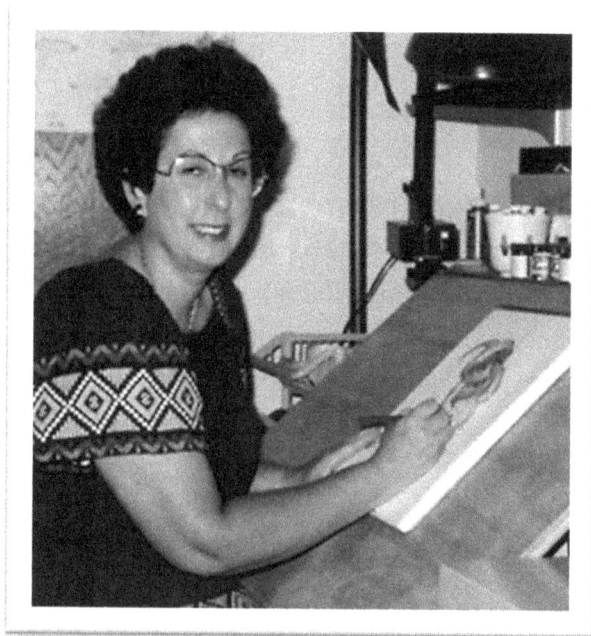

The ad using frozen waffles in place of a canvas gives endless possibilities for creative design. Nothing tells you that the waffle, syrup, honey, whipped cream, and other goodies piled on top are fattening. Why not? In this age of doctors, nutritionists, educators, and health insurers screaming that obesity leads to cancer, diabetes, heart attacks, and a host of other physical ailments, the producers of these products are not going to kill their sales by informing you about the health risks their products pose.

Women's magazines also abound with confusing messages. The cover will show a slim model or celebrity and brag about her diet and other diets to improve your health. Inside the magazine will be ads for diet supplements, diet groups, and fattening treats like pizza, strudel, cupcakes, pies, and macaroni and cheese.

Celebrities hawking diets on television, the internet, and in magazines use every trick available to make themselves look slimmer, including body shapers and other figure-constricting garments and black, dark gray, navy, and dark green clothes. These are the same tricks I used to camouflage my weight when I was obese; most people never guessed how very heavy I was. If all the celebrities were as proud of their figures as I am of mine and wanted to show them off, they would do like I do. They would throw out their figure-constricting undergarments and wear bright colors and prints. Because I am now proud of my figure, I no longer need to hide it.

Magazines tempt readers with pictures and recipes of fattening treats. Underneath each recipe is the number of calories, fat, cholesterol, carbs, fiber, protein, and sodium per serving. If I had to check out all those numbers, I would become so frustrated I would binge eat. That's too much work for me. Magazines also have ads for pre-packaged muffins, lasagna, cupcakes, candy, pizza, shakes, and spaghetti and meatballs. Advertisers claim these prepared foods are designed to help you lose weight. I am Mrs. Average. My husband and I combined do not begin to earn in a lifetime what these celebrity diet hawkers earn in one year. Diets like these may work for Miss Celebrity, who has someone in her kitchen to put the food on her table and make sure she does not eat more than the specified portion. I have never lost weight on anything that was pre-packaged. I need my meals prepared fresh.

Twenty years ago I gave up drinking fruit juices. I used to drink orange juice at breakfast and cranberry juice at lunch, mid-afternoon, at dinner, and before I went to bed. My primary care doctor said, "With your weight ballooning I want you to give up drinking all those fruit juices; they're full of sugar." After I gave up drinking juices, I switched to eating fresh fruit and picked up other vices that continued to make my weight spiral. Recently CNBC News did an interview with California State Congressman Bill Monning. He sponsored a bill in the Senate requiring the makers of sodas, fruit drinks, energy drinks, and sports drinks to put labels on their products warning people about the health risks these drinks pose. He said, "Drinking these products leads to obesity and diabetes; a 20 ounce bottle has 16 teaspoons of sugar in it."

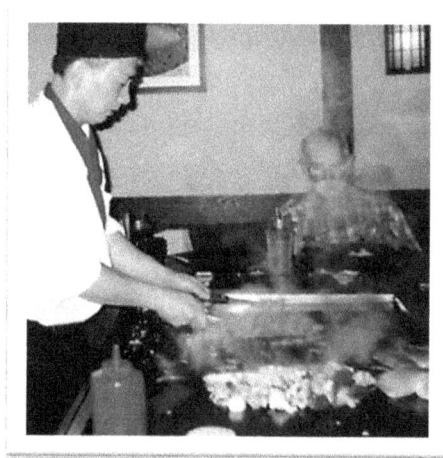

Time magazine's health section said, "Sweet Sacrifice – New guidelines seek to curb our sugar intake. . . .NO NEED TO SUGAR COAT IT: According to the new guidelines from the World Health Organization (WHO), only 5% of a person's total daily calories should come from added sugar (about 26g per day for a 2,000 calorie diet). . . .The main culprit isn't even sweets – it's processed foods. A tablespoon of ketchup has 4g sugar, a frozen pizza 26g, 1 can of tomato soup 30g, 1 blueberry muffin 22g, 1 5.7 oz. serving of orange chicken 22g, 1 cup of pasta sauce 20g sugar, and 1 cup coleslaw 23g of sugar." WOW! Sugar is everywhere, most notably in places you would never think to find it.

I believe that the subconscious mind sends messages to your brain that can derail any diet. My parents repeatedly said, "Don't do as I do, do as I say." No child, including me, does everything their parents tell them to do. My stepmother and her side of the family were thin. It seemed that they could eat anything they wanted and never gain an ounce. So I got the subliminal message that it was all right to eat what I wanted and I could eat as much as I wanted. On Sundays we visited my stepmother's relatives. On the drive from Cleveland to Euclid, Ohio we stopped at Dorsel's diner. My stepsister and I had hamburgers with all the trimmings, French fries, and chocolate milk, a drink loaded with more Hershey's Chocolate Syrup than one finds on today's sundaes. At dinner we had turkey or roast beef with either canned or package-mix gravy, stuffing, mashed potatoes loaded with sour cream and butter and topped with gravy, canned vegetables, garden salad, biscuits with butter, chocolate milk, and several pies topped with Reddy Whip or cakes topped with mounds of sugary frosting. When one of us had a birthday, chocolate or strawberry ice cream topped with chopped walnuts, chocolate syrup, and whipped cream was served.

In the late 1950's, McDonalds, Arby's, Kentucky Fried Chicken, and frozen dinners made their appearance in Cleveland. After my stepmother came back from doing the weekly grocery shopping at Fishers or Kroger's supermarkets, fast food from one of these establishments would appear on our dinner table. In addition to the fried chicken, roast beef sandwiches, or Big Mack's with coleslaw and French fries or mashed potatoes and gravy, my stepmother would put a frozen macaroni and cheese casserole in the oven. Dinner ended with apple strudel or some other form of pie or cake from Kroger's bakery counter. After meals like this, my stepmother would harp that I was too fat and needed to do something about it. With meals like this served on a regular basis, her words went in one ear and out the other.

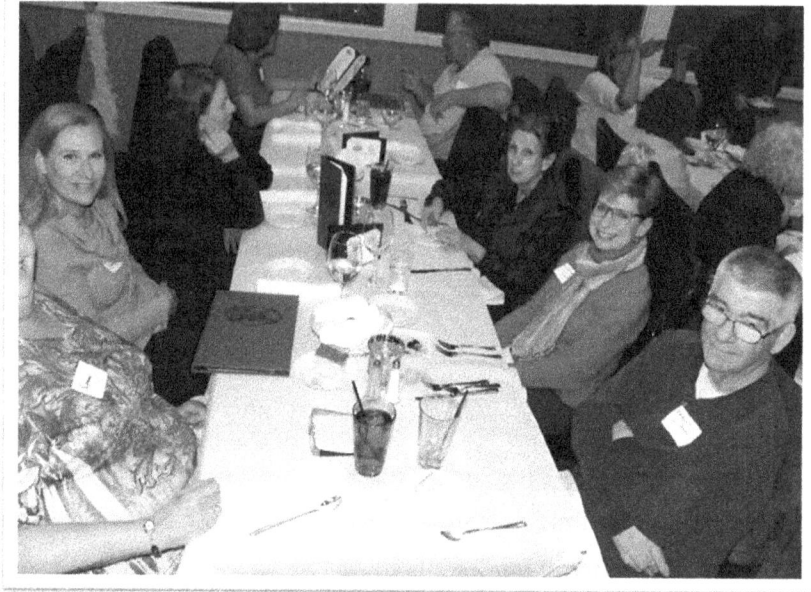

Photo courtesy of Yvonne Cunningham, organizer of ABQ Foodies
Albuquerque, NM

My father and his side of the family were more than pleasingly plump. When we visited his aunts in Kitchener, Ontario, breakfast always began with chocolate covered cream puffs and apple juice. It was followed by French toast, waffles, or pancakes with fresh whipped butter and maple syrup, baked cinnamon apples, and chocolate milk. The dining room table was piled high with little Russian cakes, cookies, and candies that one could help himself or herself to all day long. Because his aunts looked upon us as "honored guests", the lunch and dinner table was piled high with foods from the old country. I saw my great aunts' swollen legs and the difficulty they had walking, but I ignored the fact that they were overweight. Because no one in the 1940's and 1950's in my family talked about pain or their illnesses, I thought my great aunts condition was the result of being old. I never connected it to the huge quantities of fattening foods they ate. Because illnesses related to being overweight did not show up until my father's family was all senior citizens, I got the message that being fat could not harm me. As I saw it, the only harmful effect obesity caused was that my peers teased me in school and I could not find the fashionable clothes I wanted to wear at the posh department stores on Cleveland's Public Square where all my contemporaries shopped for the smart outfits they wore.

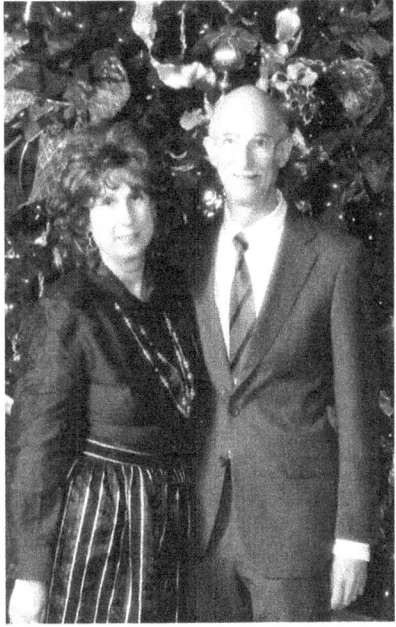

New Year's Party
Fort Worth, TX

Medical professionals did not convince me that being overweight was harmful to my health. After my children were born, doctors told me to lose weight. When I went into doctors' offices I saw doctors, nurses, receptionists, and billing clerks with their bulging thighs hanging over the edge of chairs, their lopsided walks as they shifted their bulk from side to side, and the brown bag lunches open on their desks containing cupcakes, pies, slices of cake, candy and other fattening goodies. Since they were healthcare professionals, I picked up the message that the only thing wrong with being obese was the way I looked.

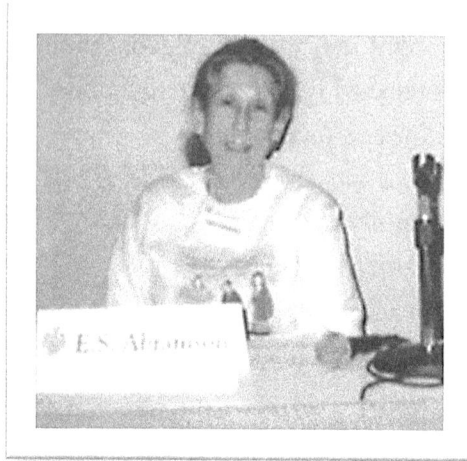

Killer Nashville crime writers' author's panel
Nashville, TN

It wasn't until my husband and I visited Casa Loma in Toronto, Ontario that I really began to understand the problems being overweight can cause. When I married Stan in 1977, he weighed 135 pounds and was 5 feet 10 inches tall. By 1996 he had gained ten pounds, but he was still thin. In 1996, I was 5 feet 4 inches tall and weighed 240 pounds. A steep staircase leads from the sidewalk up to Casa Loma's grounds. Stan walked up the stairs with ease. I huffed and puffed and barely made it to the top. I was so winded I had to sit down before we took the tour of the castle. By the time we left I was in severe pain and ready for a long nap. When we returned home, the orthopedic surgeon said I had pulled the ligaments in my knee and there was water on it. He called it "skiers' knee". He did not drain my knee. He was afraid I would have an allergic reaction because I have numerous allergies. So I spent the next year in therapy developing one reaction after another to the pain killers and creams and lotions the therapists used on my knees. I also tried every diet I heard of. The result was that they frustrated me so much I packed on more pounds.

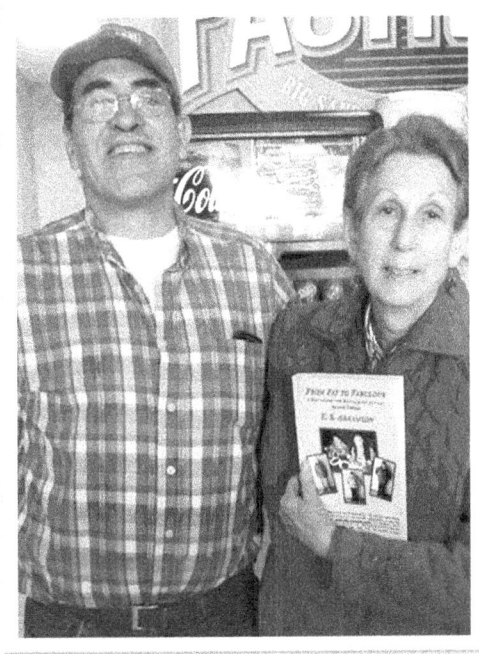

Photo courtesy of Joe Rodriguez, restaurant owner Albuquerque, NM

I am all for exercise programs for people who can and want to do them. For me, it was a disaster. Maybe it was because I did not begin an exercise program until I was in my mid-forties. While I was recuperating from DES cancer, my gynecologist and primary care doctors recommended that I exercise as a way to lessen the pain. The first program I tried was Jazzercise. I attended the one-hour sessions three times a week. At the end of five months I lost thirty pounds and two dress sizes. But I also threw my back out. The pain was almost as bad as when I had had a slipped disk twenty years earlier. For the next six months I shuffled around the house holding onto walls, ate everything in the refrigerator, and gained fifty pounds.

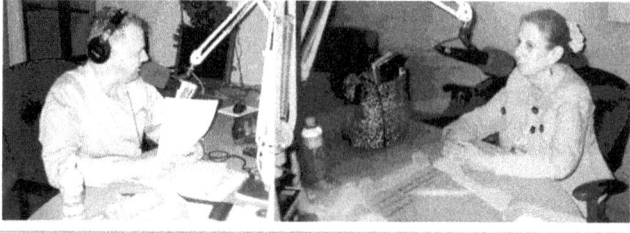

Food Talk STL, 590-AM Radio KFNS

Jazzercise was followed by the YWCA's water aerobics program for people with arthritis. It was billed as low-impact exercise for people who could not do strenuous exercises. I not only did not lose any weight, I ended up gaining weight by going out to eat with my fellow classmates. We chowed down at the local fast-food restaurants and talked about the fabulous fashions we had seen in women's magazines. All of us hoped to lose enough weight and proportions to get into them. None of us achieved our goal.

After the YWCA I tried the more strenuous water aerobics program at The Q. On this program too I continued to gain weight and proportions. I was so tired and stressed out from the sessions that the minute I got home I raided the refrigerator.

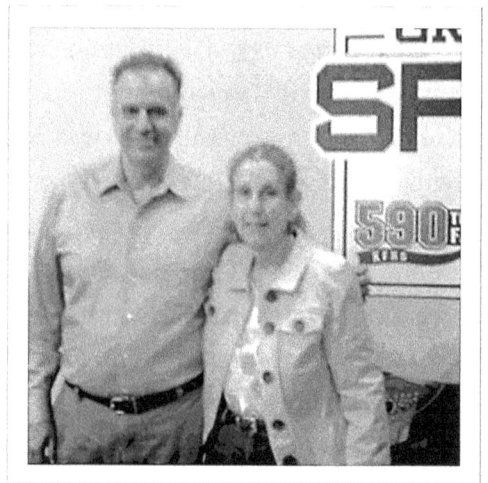

Photo courtesy of David Craig, Food Talk STL, 590-AM Radio KFNS

Today I do only low-impact aerobics. I walk a dog and ride an old-fashioned stationary exercise bike. Because I am never hungry on my restaurant lover's diet, I do not need to raid the refrigerator even after walking the dog or riding my bike.

Prior to beginning my restaurant lovers' diet, I compared my walk to that of an overstuffed penguin. I waddled. My knees sank under my weight. In my sixties, doctors claimed that I would never walk again if I didn't have a knee replacement operation. During the first year on my restaurant lovers' diet I shed fifty pounds. The second year I lost another thirty-five pounds. The third year I lost another twenty pounds. To date, I have lost one hundred pounds. I credit my restaurant lovers' diet with giving me back my life. I have not had knee replacement surgery and I am doing things I could only dream of doing previously.

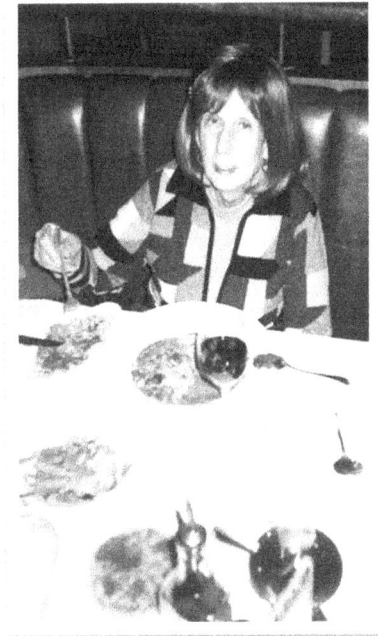

St. Louis Branch
National League of
American Pen Women's
Dinner

From birth until the age of six, I was a skinny child. After my spleen was removed my family was so worried I would not survive that they encouraged me to eat. In the 1940's we did not have the proliferation of microwavable hot and cold cereals that you shake out of the box into a bowl and add milk to that we have today, nor did we have the frozen waffles, pancakes, biscuits and gravy, and egg, ham, and cheese sandwiches. Mothers stood over gas stoves cooking breakfast for their children. My stepmother prepared Cream of Wheat with butter, brown sugar, raisins, and honey. Because we did not have a toaster, bread was toasted in the oven. A glass of freshly squeezed orange juice and a glass of whole milk were served with it. When I was eight, my stepmother and I got into a heated argument. I don't remember what it was about, but whatever it was, it must have been a whopper because from that day on, she never again got up to make my breakfast. Left to my own devices and needing to grab something quickly so I would not be late for school, I raided the refrigerator and ate leftover sweet rolls, cold spaghetti, and hamburger, salami, baloney, and pastrami sandwiches. I do not know if this incident is where my dislike of traditional breakfast food began, but to this day I do not eat traditional breakfast foods. As for lunch, I packed whatever could be stuffed quickly into a brown bag. Good nutrition was the last thing on my mind.

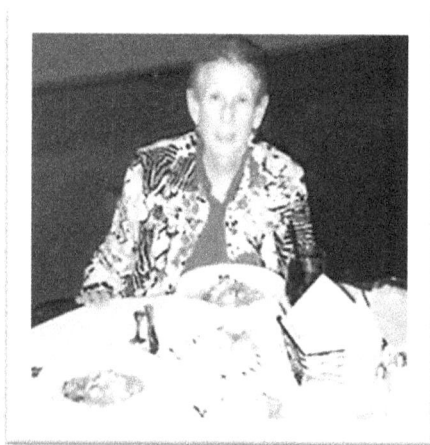

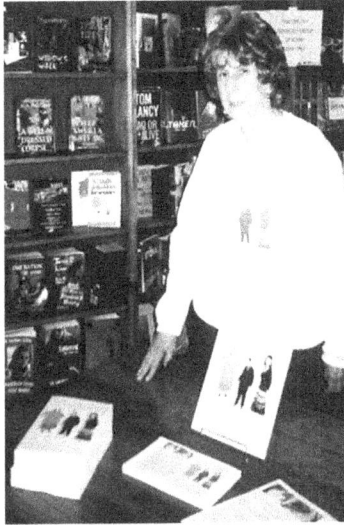

Photo courtesy of All On The Same
Page bookstore

I ate lunch with my paternal grandmother every Saturday. Shortly after I arrived at her apartment, we walked hand in hand down to the corner deli. After she had the deli counterman slice a pound of Vienna kosher baloney and a fresh rye bread, we added Wise Potato Chips, Cotton Club cherry soda, and a cake to the basket, then checked out. Back at her apartment, we spread the feast out on the enameled kitchen table and ate with gusto. The feast was always followed by cherry Jell-O and strawberry candy. I looked forward to those Saturdays never realizing what all that junk food was doing to my body.

In the 1950's all the girls wore pencil-slim skirts that were so straight and tight they could barely move. The 90 to 100 pound feminine beauties wore clothes I could only dream about. I was the 5-foot-4-inch165-pound teenager everyone made fun of because of her size. To minimize my rotund appearance, I took out my sewing machine and made skirts and dresses with full skirts.

In *From Fat to Fabulous: A Diet Guide for Restaurant Lovers* and *We Went From Fat to Fabulous: A Diet Guide for Restaurant Lovers* I related the story of Gail and her inability to lose weight. Because readers continue to ask if Gail ever took off the weight, I am updating Gail's story.

Sad to say, every time I see Gail, she appears to have gained more weight. Chairs sag under her, she waddles when she walks, and she can no longer bend over and see her feet. She opts to sit at a table with sturdy wooden chairs at our writing group's favorite Italian restaurant instead of sitting in a booth. And she continues to cry about her struggle to take off pounds.

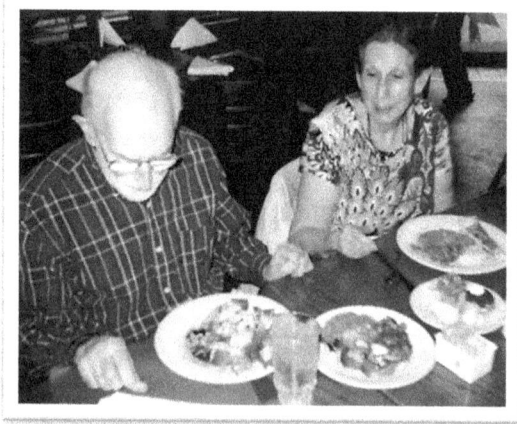

After the tall blonde waitress with gray streaks in her hair, who mopped sweat from her brow on her t-shirt sleeve, took everyone's order, it was my turn. When I ordered minestrone soup, a garden salad without croutons or cucumbers and creamy Italian dressing, chicken Marsala without any breading or flour, green beans and ice tea without any ice, Gail's eyes bulged out.

"You're going to eat all that?" she asked.

"Yes," I replied.

"And you claim you're on a diet?"

"I am."

The waitress, with a pencil poised over her notepad, nodded in Gail's direction. "What'll you have, Hon?"

"I'll have a garden salad with extra croutons, and I'll have her croutons too." Gail looked at me. "And an order of toasted ravioli and a diet soda."

The moment the waitress left our table to place the group's order, Mary tapped me on the shoulder. "Did you see that? She ordered double croutons and took yours too."

"Yes," I whispered.

The waitress placed a basket of bread and pats of butter on the table. Gail scooped the basket up in her arms and began tearing the loaf of Italian bread apart. She made her usual concoction of butter, olive oil, and grated parmesan cheese, dunked the bread in it, and began eating. "I can't get bread this good at home," she said.

Jenny signaled the waitress for another basket of bread. When it arrived, she placed it at her end of the table out of Gail's reach.

Gail ate half of her salad and half of the ravioli, and then signaled the waitress to have the remainder of her salad, ravioli, and marinara sauce wrapped up. "I'm too full. I'm going to save the rest for my dinner."

Mary tapped me on the shoulder again. "Full? Right! After three loaves of bread I would be full too."

If I had eaten the amount of bread, croutons, ravioli, and diet soda that Gail ate that day, I would never have lost any weight. I cannot stress it enough, _no_ diet, mine included, will work if you cheat.

Yogurt commercials brag that their products contain only 80 to 90 tiny calories. They show slim happy people eating yogurt for breakfast, lunch, snacks, and dessert. In 1976 after my marriage to my first husband Bernard was annulled by the religious court, I became the sole support of two minor children and a dog. It was also the year that the bottom fell out of the home crafts market. I had been designing latchhook rug kits for Rapco and other crafts companies, but now I was out of a job. It took several months before I found employment at Montgomery Wards selling sewing machines and teaching women how to use them. During the period between jobs, Bernard refused to give me or the children any money for food or the other necessities of life. My attorney advised me to apply for welfare. Because I needed to watch every penny, during this period I developed my yogurt diet. I ate one carton of yogurt for breakfast, one for lunch, and one for dinner and gave all the other food in the refrigerator and cupboards to my children to prevent them from starving. My stomach growled "feed me", and I had headaches resulting from hunger all the time. In less than six months I lost 100 pounds and went from a size 24w to having clothes donated to me by my friends' slender teenage daughters. Welfare doctors never asked about my diet. They just assumed that such a great weight loss in such a short period of time was due to cancer. I wound up being rushed into Baltimore's Sinai Hospital for a biopsy for breast cancer. When the biopsy revealed that I did not have cancer, the doctors scratched their heads and suggested other unprovable reasons for my drastic weight loss. In spite of the fact that all the doctors in that section of the hospital treated only welfare patients, none of them ever considered diet as a factor. When I was gainfully employed again, I put the weight back on faster than I had taken it off.

I have read numerous studies that claim overweight women have poor relationships with their mothers. For a while I thought that might be the reason I was obese, so I tried mending the fences. All it did was leave me more frustrated than I already was, and I ate more to compensate for my inability to have what I thought should be a normal mother-daughter relationship.

After I married Stan, my second husband, we threw out all the canned, packaged, and frozen foods in the house. He did not want any food in the house with preservatives in it. All foods had to be fresh. When I prepared a meal, I stood over the stove tasting everything to make sure it was just right. What I didn't realize was that all that tasting was expanding my waistline.

The FDA limits the amount of rodent droppings, maggots, rodent hairs and other appetite suppressants in processed foods, but that limit is <u>not</u> zero. Supposedly those disgusting things are not harmful to your health. Just the thought of it is enough to send me to the nearest lavatory to vomit. On the other hand, restaurants are inspected by city and county health inspectors. If they find revolting stuff like that in the food, they shut the establishment down. It cannot reopen until it passes another inspection. Now you know why I avoid all processed food, opting for freshly prepared restaurant meals instead.

Many dentists refer to sucrose (sugar) as "a toxin or a poison". They also include high fructose corn syrup in this description noting that it is often the underlying cause of obesity, diabetes, Alzheimer's, tooth decay, skin problems, and a host of other diseases.

As an artist, I am fascinated by findings related to art. It is interesting to note that dentists study the paintings hanging in art museums. They discovered that prior to 1700, paintings depicted happy, smiling people; but after 1700, portraits commissioned by the upper classes showed them with their mouths closed. The reason for that was sugar consumption had decayed their teeth, turning them an ugly black/brown. Because the importation of sugar was so expensive until the 1800's when it decreased in cost, only the wealthy could afford it. When it became affordable in the 1800's, tooth decay became the common man's problem too.

What I am about to say is <u>not</u> to be taken as medical advice. It is strictly to inform you that sugar can be found in the most unlikely places. In *We Went From Fat to Fabulous: A Diet Guide for Restaurant Lovers* I wrote about having worked for a manufacturer of generic drugs. I mentioned that my weighing room partner and I measured sugar for drug coatings. I also said that sugar coatings cover drugs to counteract their bitterness and make them easier to swallow.

Recently I had a very severe sinus infection. My primary care doctor prescribed antibiotics and Mucusinex, a chest congestion expectorant. I said I had been taking two pills per day of a drug store's generic brand of mucus relief. The pharmacist had told me that it had the same drug composition as the name brand drug. She said, "That's true, but you have to take twice as much because only the name brand holds the patent for the long lasting mucus relief drug. So, you have to take four a day instead of two." I went home and for the first time since I got sick checked my weight on my digital scale. I had gained a pound. My doctor's explanation about the generic brand versus the name brand made it easy for me to see where the extra sugar in my diet had come from. You are probably saying to yourself "What's one pound? It's nothing to get upset over." I thought about the one pound I gained on the generic drug and concluded that if generic drugs caused me to gain one pound over the period of one week, at the end of the year I would have gained fifty-two pounds. I immediately rushed out to the drugstore and purchased the name brand medicine.

The Earl of Sandwich did not do our waistlines any favors when he invented the sandwich in 1762. History records that John Montagu, the fourth Earl of Sandwich, had his hands full as First Sea Lord commanding the British Navy and as a dedicated gambler with a love of day-long card games. This led to little time for eating. His idea for the sandwich came up at the card table. He had waiters put pieces of meat between two slices of bread so he wouldn't get his fingers greasy while he played. From then on it did not matter if he was fighting great sea battles or laying down a Royal Flush; he could eat food without much fuss. Today the sandwich is the world's most popular fast food. Like canned, frozen, and other processed foods, it contains huge amounts of carbohydrates and refined sugars that make waistlines bulge and scales groan.

Stan and I ate at a lovely little family-run Mexican restaurant on the US Mexican border. The owner and her daughters were all more

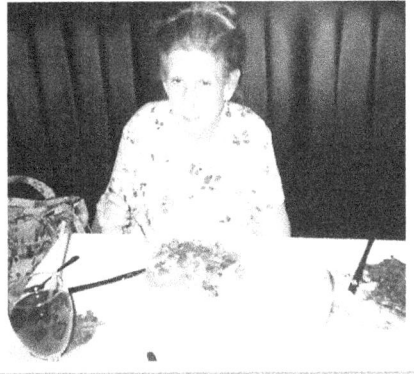

than pleasingly plump. Immediately after we sat down, a basket of tortilla chips and salsa were put on the table. We ordered the beef and chicken fajitas for lunch. Our order came with grilled beef and chicken, onions, red and green peppers, refried beans, Spanish rice, grilled corn, and flour tortillas. A side dish contained shredded lettuce, diced tomatoes, sour cream, shredded cheddar cheese, and guacamole. While we were eating, our waitress placed a basket of sopaillas and a bottle of honey on the table. Before she handed us our check, she asked if we wanted dessert. A meal like this is a recipe for a diet disaster. It is all right to eat tortilla chips, corn, rice, beans, guacamole, tortillas, and sopaillas with honey on reward nights; but even then, all of them should not be eaten at the same time. Select two of these at most.

As with any diet, mine included, you still need some form of exercise. To this day I still walk a dog and ride a stationary bike. _No diet_, mine included, will succeed if you cheat.

There are very few rules to my restaurant lover's diet. When traveling I pass up the free breakfasts provided by hotels because I do not eat hot or cold cereal, sausages, bacon, ham, toast, bagels, donuts, pastry, waffles, powdered eggs, or hash brown potatoes. AOL's travel writer claims "Hotels Serve Glorified Prison Food For Breakfast. I've never been to a prison, but I can't help but wonder if convicts get nicer breakfasts than what you find on the breakfast buffets at most American chain hotels these days." I only stay at hotels where I can have a refrigerator and microwave in my room so I can eat my previous night's restaurant leftovers.

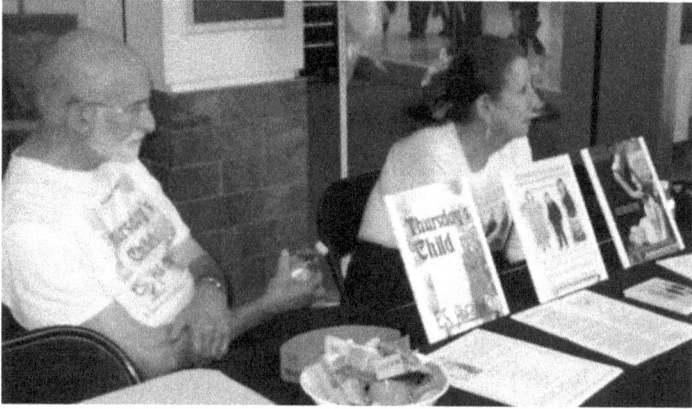

Photo courtesy of Pam DeVoe, past president of Sisters in Crime, St. Louis, MO

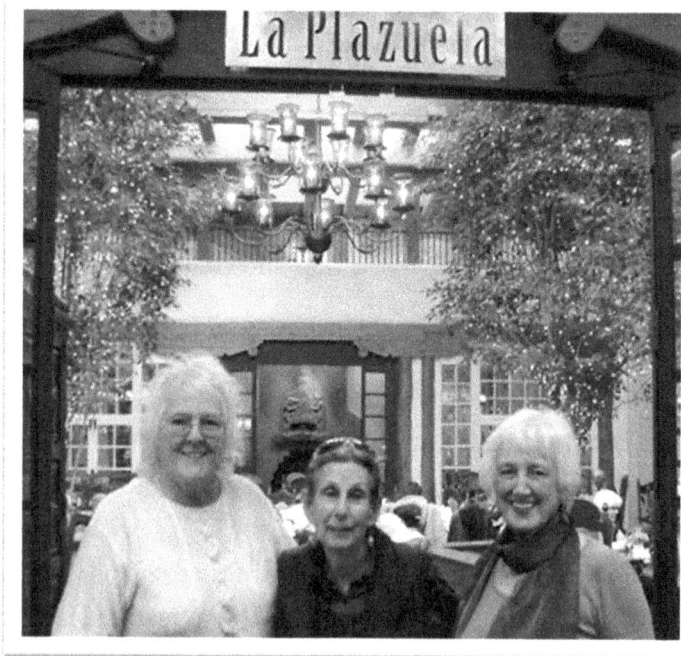

Photo courtesy of Jane Maclean, past president of the Albuquerque, NM branch of the National League of American Pen Women

Most restaurants will be happy to make changes if you request them. I do not eat any bread, bacon, ham, shellfish, fish or American cheese and do not drink soda. I eat pasta, pizza, potatoes, rice, beans or dessert on reward nights. After the National Institute for Health reported that rice and products made from rice, such as cereals and snacks, contain arsenic that is derived from the soil, I have severely limited the amount of rice I eat. NIH has also reported that potatoes derive nicotine from the soil. The bread part can be a little tricky. Because menus often do not say that meat, vegetables, soups, or cheeses are coated with flour, tapioca starch, matzo meal, potato starch, corn starch or bread crumbs, before ordering I always ask the waitperson if the food is prepared with them. When I order French onion soup, I ask the waitperson to tell the chef to leave out the bread and croutons. I order all salads without bacon, cucumbers, and croutons. With veal, chicken, and eggplant, I ask them to not use any breading or flour. I do not eat the bread or tortillas the waitperson puts on the table. I ask that all my food be prepared fresh. I do not want it frozen, prepackaged, or from boxes because food prepared in these manners often contain bread products and excessively large amounts of salt and sugar. These are the cheap fillers that made me fat. I trim every scrap of fat off my meat. That includes removing the skin from chicken and turkey. I never add salt or sugar to my food. I drink lots of regular or decaffeinated coffee or herbal tea with a low-calorie sweetener or I drink water. My husband and I share appetizers, side salads, and soups. Flatbreads, pizzas, quesadillas, and pasta are only eaten on reward nights. When we order a dessert on a reward night, we share it too. Both of us order our own main course.

I order _all_ sandwiches open-faced. I have an aversion to fat and grease. I tried having   restaurants leave off the bread or bun and use a paper towel to drain off the fat and grease, but that left the meat dry and tasteless. I like my meat juicy. I finally realized that since I do not eat the bread, I could use it to soak up the fat and grease, so I started having my sandwiches served open-faced.

Chocolate is the food of the gods. I am a chocoholic. No diet on this earth will ever make me give up my chocolate fix. My refrigerator is never without a supply of Lindt Excellence Intense Orange Dark Chocolate or Lindt Excellence 70% Cocoa Smooth Dark Chocolate bars. Every afternoon I eat two chocolate squares out of the ten squares or one-fifth of a 3.5 ounce bar.

All of the diets I have previously been on require the dieter to strictly follow the diet and never deviate from its rules in any way whatsoever. On my restaurant lover's diet, I give myself a reward for losing weight and inches three days per month and on special occasions. For example, on my birthday I had a glass of Lambrusco and roasted potatoes with dinner and a   large piece of decadent dark chocolate cake topped with whipped cream for dessert.

I eat until I feel full. Usually this amounts to approximately half of one entrée plus the appetizer, soup, and salad I share with my husband. I take home the remainder of my entrée. I discovered that there is a big difference in how full I feel after a meal between drinking hot and cold beverages. I try to drink beverages hot as often as possible because I feel full sooner and the feeling lasts longer. Doctors instruct you to put ice on injuries to take the pain and swelling down. Apparently ice can also numb your stomach thereby preventing you from knowing when you are full. With warm or hot drinks, I know instantly when I am full and I stop eating.

I eat a moderately sized breakfast. Lunch is my biggest meal of the day. Dinner is the smallest. I try to eat my last meal of the day at least three hours before I go to bed.

For breakfast, in _all_ restaurants I choose one entrée plus decaffeinated coffee or hot tea with a low calorie sweetener.

For lunch or dinner, in _all_ restaurants I choose one appetizer, one soup, and one side salad to share with my husband. I order my own entrée and either iced tea without ice or hot tea with a low calorie sweetener. He drinks water or wine with dinner. When I ask the waitperson to leave off seafood or ham, most restaurants will ask if I want something in place of it. I order an extra salad or vegetable.

On reward days I choose one dessert and share it with my husband.

The restaurants mentioned in my restaurant lover's guide are here because their owners or managers gave me copies of their menus and have been gracious enough to answer my questions. Their management and wait staff are a wonderful group of men and women. In order to be in this guide, the restaurant must serve its meals on plates and provide knives and forks. The necessity for these utensils will become more obvious as you view the selections my husband and I made from the menus the restaurants provided and read my comments. The only menu selections that appear in *From Fat to Fabulous: A Diet Guide for Restaurant Lover* are the foods that my husband and I eat. We have eaten at all of the establishments listed in this guide. Their menus are arranged in alphabetical order.

I hope you enjoy my restaurant diet as much as I do.

Happy eating,
Elaine

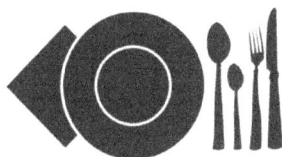

THE RESTAURANTS

BREAKFAST

Basil's Kitchen & Bar/Hilton
Chain Restaurant

Hilton Breakfast Buffet:

Featuring fresh seasonal fruits, eggs any style and omelets prepared to order, assorted cheeses and meats, fresh juices, milk, coffee and more...

A La Carte Breakfast Menu:

Breakfast Specialties:

Breakfast Wrap – Scrambled eggs with grilled onions, peppers, sausage and cheddar cheese in a warm flour tortilla, served with breakfast potatoes. I ask the waitperson to ask the chef to substitute extra grilled onions and peppers for the sausage and potatoes.

Omelets – Three eggs lightly seasoned, filled with your choice of ingredients, served with breakfast potatoes and your choice of bacon or sausage and your favorite toasted bread. I ask the waitperson to ask the chef to substitute extra vegetables and cheese for the bacon, potatoes, and bread.

Sides and Beverages:

Fresh Fruit

Fresh Brewed Coffee

Hot Tea – Assorted and herbal varieties.

Chilled Juices – Choices include orange, cranberry, and apple.

Chilled Milk

Hot Chocolate – I drink hot chocolate on a reward day.

Mimi's Café
Chain Restaurant

Quiche, Crepes & More:

With fresh-cut fruit.

All-Butter Croissant Egg & Bacon Sandwich – Two fried eggs, sliced tomatoes, melted cheddar cheese and hickory-smoked bacon. With a side of Dijon mustard. I ask the waitperson to ask the chef to scramble my eggs and to substitute extra tomatoes for the bacon.

Chef's Choice Quiche

Egg, Spinach & Cheese Crepes – Tomatoes, onions and a drizzle of creamy Monroy cheese sauce.

Omelets:

With toast or muffin, and potatoes roasted with savory thyme & basil. I eat the potatoes or the muffin, but not both.

Hickory-Smoked Ham & Cheese – Red and green bell peppers, caramelized onions and cheddar cheese. I ask the waitperson to ask the chef to substitute extra bell peppers for the ham.

Egg White & Veggie – Open-faced egg white omelet with spinach, mushrooms, caramelized onions, tomatoes and goat cheese. With fresh-cut fruit (no potatoes).

Farmhouse Two-Egg Breakfasts:

With toast or muffin, and potatoes roasted with savory thyme & basil. I eat the potatoes or the muffin, but not both.

Turkey Sausage & Eggs

Corned Beef Hash & Eggs

Eggs

Pueblo Harvest Café & Bakery
Indian Cultural Center
Albuquerque, NM

Breakfast: Served 8a to 11a

Build Your Own Pueblo Breakfast – Served with Pueblo Beans and Breakfast Potatoes. I ask the waitperson to substitute fruit for the beans and potatoes. I eat the meals with Fritos, cornmeal, bread or fry bread on a reward day.

Choose your eggs.

Choose your meat – 3 chili turkey sausage.

Choose your bread – oven bread, fry bread, handmade tortilla.

Pueblo Eggs Benedict – Two towers of grilled oven bread with seasonal sliced heirloom tomatoes, 3 chili turkey sausage and your choice of eggs. Smothered with homemade Benedict sauce. Served with grilled asparagus.

Breakfast Yogurt Parfait – Layers of homemade granola, Greek style yogurt, and fresh fruit finished with New Mexico honey.

Albuquerque Morning – A breakfast sandwich served on grilled oven bread with scrambled eggs, 3 chili turkey sausage and cheddar cheese.

Chackewe con Huevos – Traditional blue cornmeal topped with carne adovada, two eggs cooked any style, cheddar cheese and fresh diced tomatoes. I ask the waitperson to ask the chef to substitute turkey for the carne adovada.

Breakfast Frito Pie – A layer of Fritos covered with ground 3 chili turkey sausage, two eggs cooked any style, green chili sauce, cheddar cheese, freshly diced tomatoes and onions.

Denver Omelet – Three egg omelet with cheddar Jack cheese, sautéed mushrooms, bell peppers, sautéed onion and diced ham. I ask the waitperson to ask the chef to substitute turkey for the ham.

ABQ Omelet – Three egg omelet with Pepper Jack cheese, diced Bueno Green Chili®, heirloom tomatoes, sautéed onions and 3- chili turkey sausage. Smothered with your choice of chili.

A La Carte

Chili

Cup or fruit

Eggs

Meat (3 chili turkey sausage)

Side of asparagus or heirloom tomatoes

Schneithorst
Ladue, MO

Steak and Eggs -A 9 ounce strip steak with two eggs, hash browns and toast. I ask the waitperson to ask the chef to substitute fruit for the hash browns and toast.

Make Your Own Breakfast Sandwich – Two eggs, your choice of cheese, meat and bread with hash browns. I ask the waitperson to ask the chef to substitute fruit for the bread and hash browns.

Three Egg Omelet – Your choice of any three: bacon, ham, sausage, mushrooms, onions, spinach, green peppers, tomatoes, cheese. Served with choice of toast and hash browns. I chose from the mushrooms, onions, spinach, green peppers, tomatoes or cheese and ask the waitperson to ask the chef to substitute fruit for the hash browns and toast.

A La Carte:

Fresh Fruit Bowl

Turkey Patties – Two patties.

One Egg

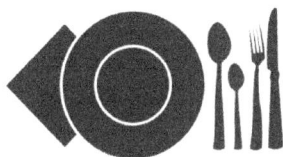

The Restaurants

Lunch and Dinner

Bandana's
Chain Restaurant

Sandwiches:

Served on our signature grilled Bandana's bun with your choice of one regular side.

> Beef Sandwich
>
> Pulled Chicken Sandwich
>
> Turkey Sandwich

Platters:

Served with garlic bread and your choice of two regular sides. I do not eat the garlic bread. Dinner portions are 9 oz. of meat and lunch portions are 6 oz. of meat.

> Beef Platter
>
> Chicken Platter
>
> Turkey Platter

Combination Platters:

Served with garlic bread and your choice of two regular sides. I do not eat the garlic bread. Choose 2 portions that are 6 oz. each of meat or choose 3 portions that are 5 oz. of meat each. Beef, Chicken, or Turkey.

Salads, Spuds & Tenders:

> Bar-B-Q Salad – Salad greens with beef, turkey, or chicken. Ranch dressing or bar-b-q ranch dressing.

Starters:

> Brunswick Stew

Side Orders:

Cole Slaw

Green Beans

Dinner Salad

Basil's Kitchen & Bar/Hilton
Chain Restaurant

"A taste of the Mediterranean". Our cuisine features fresh pastas, steak dishes and several fat-free and low curb dishes prepared with fresh herbs. We pride ourselves on the highest quality of food and exceptional service for your dining experience. If there is something you would like, just ask. We are here to serve you and you are always welcome at Basil's."

Lunch Menu:

"A taste of the Mediterranean"

Appetizers:

<u>Antipasti Plate</u> – Prosciutto di Parma, salami, mortadella and roasted tomatoes with fresh mozzarella, olives and grissini bread sticks. I ask the waitperson to ask the chef to substitute extra roasted tomatoes for the prosciutto and grissini bread sticks.

<u>Roasted Garlic, Spinach, and Artichoke Dip</u> – Served warm with corn tortilla chips.

Flatbreads:

I eat flatbreads on a reward night.

<u>Pesto Chicken and Roasted Peppers</u> – Herb crusted flatbread layered with parmesan sauce, topped with pesto chicken and roasted peppers sprinkled with mozzarella cheese and baked to perfection.

<u>Margherita</u>- Marinated tomatoes, oregano, basil and mozzarella cheese on herb crusted flat bread baked to perfection.

Salads and Soup:

Northern Bean Soup – White beans simmered with tomatoes, onions, topped with pancetta and pasta. I ask the waitperson to ask the chef to leave off the pancetta and pasta.

Basil's House Salad – Fresh Romaine and spring mix with cucumbers and cherry tomatoes, served with your choice of dressing. I ask the waitperson to ask the chef to substitute extra tomatoes for the cucumbers.

Greek Salad – Mixed greens tossed in lemon olive oil vinaigrette with an olive medley, cucumbers, and grape tomatoes topped with Bermuda onions and feta cheese. I ask the waitperson to ask the chef to substitute extra tomatoes for the cucumbers.

Spinach and Arugula Salad – Organic tender leaf spinach and arugula with portabella mushrooms, red onions, roasted tomatoes and gorgonzola cheese, topped with apple wood smoked bacon and toasted pine nuts, served with apple cider vinaigrette. Add grilled chicken or steak for an additional charge. I ask the waitperson to ask the chef to substitute extra red onions for the smoked bacon.

Basil's Grilled Black and Bleu Steak Salad – Mixed green salad tossed with caramelized onions, bleu cheese crumbles, grape tomatoes, cucumbers and house-made croutons, topped with grilled sirloin and your choice of dressing. I ask the waitperson to ask the chef to substitute extra tomatoes and mixed salad greens for the cucumbers and croutons.

Sandwiches, Burgers and More:

(Choice of fruit, French fries, zucchini fries, or pasta salad). I always order the fruit.

Vermont Cheddar Burger – 1/2 lb. fresh Angus beef grilled to perfection, topped with cheddar cheese on a brioche bun.

Basil's Free Range Turkey Club Sandwich – Classic club

sandwich on a butter croissant with turkey, lettuce, smoked apple wood bacon, tomatoes, and Swiss cheese. I ask the waitperson to ask the chef to leave out the center slice of bread and to substitute extra lettuce and tomato for the bacon.

Bistecca Steak Sandwich – Marinated sirloin with caramelized onions, wild mushrooms and melted provolone on a pretzel hoagie bun.

Grilled Chicken Caprese – Herb marinated chicken breast topped with fresh tomatoes, mozzarella, and pesto mayo on a focaccia bun.

Roasted Vegetable Wrap – Fresh vegetables marinated in olive oil and Mediterranean seasonings, wrapped in a low-carb tortilla wrap. Turkey is available for an additional charge.

Dinner Menu:

For appetizers, flatbreads, salads and soups, and sandwiches, burgers and more see lunch menu.

Appetizers:

Beef Tips Cabernet – Sautéed beef tips with wild mushrooms, shallots, tomatoes and Cabernet wine sauce, finished with gorgonzola cheese.

Entrees:

Chicken Marsala Ravioli – Chicken Marsala filled ravioli tossed with pearl onions and wild mushrooms in a Marsala wine sauce, garnished with sautéed spinach. I eat Chicken Marsala Ravioli on a reward night.

Herb Roasted Springer Mountain Chicken with Lemon and Thyme – With natural jus broth, glazed in white wine, served with roasted Italian herb potatoes and grilled asparagus. I ask the waitperson to ask the chef to substitute extra grilled asparagus for the potatoes.

Basil's Filet Mignon – Grilled to perfection with a Cabernet balsamic reduction, served with sour cream and chive mashed potatoes and a vegetable medley. I ask the waitperson to ask the chef to substitute grilled asparagus for the mashed potatoes.

Bistecca Steak – Marinated grilled loin with wild mushroom risotto and grilled vegetables. I ask the waitperson to ask the chef to substitute extra grilled vegetables for the mushroom risotto.

Weekly Specials:

Flatbread – Grilled steak, caramelized onions, wild mushrooms and crumbled bleu cheese. I eat flatbread on a reward night.

Sandwich – Greek sirloin wrap with herb pasta salad. I ask the waitperson to ask the chef to substitute a mixed green salad for the pasta salad.

Salad – Southern fried chicken salad with cheddar cheese, cucumbers, grape tomatoes, pecans and served with honey mustard dressing. I ask the waitperson to ask the chef to substitute grilled chicken for the fried chicken and to substitute extra tomatoes for the cucumbers.

Dessert:

Brownie – Ala mode with sweet cream ice cream.

Charcoal House
Glendale, MO

Appetizers:

Soup du Jour

Salads:

All salads are served ala Carte.

Dinner Salad

Greek Salad

Caesar Salad – I ask the waitperson to ask the chef to leave off the croutons and to substitute bleu cheese dressing for the Caesar dressing.

Spinach Salad

Dressings: Creamed or grated Roquefort, house, or ranch.

Entrees:

All Entrees are served with choice of potato or vegetable, rolls and butter. I choose the vegetable and leave the rolls.

Tenderloin Tips – Topped with sautéed mushrooms.

Broiled Half-Chicken

Baby Loin Lamb Chops – Charbroiled and served with mint jelly. I ask the waitperson to ask the chef to leave off the mint jelly.

Chopped Sirloin Steak – Topped with sautéed mushrooms.

Gourmet Dinner for Two:

Chateaubriand – Double thick tender center cut of beef tenderloin, surrounded by vegetables and garnished with onion rings. Served with choice of potato or vegetable, dinner salad or small Caesar salad. I order the dinner salad and I ask the waiter to substitute extra vegetables for the onion rings and potato.

Beef en Brochette:

Choice pieces of beef tenderloin, green peppers, tomato, mushrooms and onion cooked on a skewer and served on a bed of rice. I ask the waitperson to ask the chef to substitute extra vegetables for the rice.

Steaks:

All steaks are charcoal broiled (unless otherwise specified). For something different – try a steak smothered with toasted Roquefort cheese! All steaks include choice of potato or vegetable, rolls and butter. I ask the waitperson to ask the chef to substitute a vegetable for the potato. I do not eat the rolls.

Charcoal House Special – Center cut filet mignon topped with sautéed mushrooms.

Steak by George – Center cut filet mignon garnished with onion rings. I ask the waitperson to ask the chef to substitute a vegetable for the onion rings.

Extra Large Filet Mignon – Topped with sautéed mushrooms.

New York Cut Sirloin Strip

Gourmet Special Sirloin Strip – Garnished with onion rings. I ask the waitperson to ask the chef to substitute a vegetable for the onion rings.

Extra Large Sirloin Strip

T-bone – 21 oz.

Desserts:

Chocolate Cake

Chili's Grill & Bar
International Chain Restaurant

Appetizers:

All of our appetizers are made to order and deliver big flavor that's simply too good not to share.

Skillet Queso – Cheese dip with seasoned beef. Served with warm tostada chips and salsa.

Hot Spinach & Artichoke Dip – Blend of Romano, cream cheese, mozzarella, parmesan, chopped spinach and artichokes, freshly baked and topped with house made pico de gallo. Served with tostada chips.

Margherita Flatbread – Classic with a definite southwest accent. Topped with Monterey Jack, mozzarella, roasted garlic aioli & fresh tomatoes with a drizzle of cilantro-ranch pesto.

California Grilled Chicken Flatbread – Topped with grilled chicken, Applewood smoked bacon, tomato sauce, Monterey Jack, mozzarella, chopped cilantro, house made pico de gallo, fresh sliced avocado, and a drizzle of roasted garlic aioli. I ask the waitperson to ask the chef to substitute extra Monterey Jack for the bacon and avocado.

Chipotle Chicken Flatbread – Topped with grilled chili-rubbed chicken, tomato sauce, cheddar, Monterey Jack, mozzarella, chopped cilantro, house made pico de gallo & a drizzle chipotle pesto.

Soups, Chili & Salad:

Warm your taste buds with our flavorful soups and world-famous chili or try one of our delicious sides.

House Salad – With croutons, tomatoes, red onions, cucumbers, and cheese. Served with your choice of dressing. I ask the waitperson to ask the chef to substitute extra tomatoes and red onions for the cucumbers and the croutons.

Soup & House Salad – A delicious bowl of soup with a House Salad with your choice of dressing. See House Salad above.

Chicken Caesar Salad – Grilled breast of chicken, parmesan and garlic croutons with creamy Caesar dressing. I ask the waitperson to ask the chef to substitute extra romaine lettuce for the croutons and to substitute blue cheese dressing for the Caesar dressing.

Chicken Enchilada Soup – Topped with tortilla strips and 3-cheese blend. I ask the waitperson to ask the chef to leave off the tortilla strips.

Chili & House Salad – A delicious bowl of chili with a House Salad with your choice of dressing.

Southwest Chicken Soup – Oven roasted chicken, hominy & tomato in flavorful ancho-chili chicken broth. Topped with crispy tortilla strips and chopped cilantro. I ask the waitperson to ask the chef to leave off the tortilla strips.

Santa Fe Chicken Salad – Grilled chili-rubbed chicken with spicy Santa Fe sauce, house made pico de gallo, fresh diced avocado, chopped cilantro, crispy tortilla strips with house-made ranch dressing. I ask the waitperson to ask the chef to substitute extra pico de gallo for the avocado and the tortilla strips.

Trilingual Chili – Slow-cooked chili with beef, onions, and chilies. Topped with cheese.

Caribbean Salad – Fresh hand-cut pineapple, mandarin oranges, dried cranberries, diced red bell peppers, chopped green onions, cilantro and sesame seeds with a honey-lime dressing. Chicken can be added for an additional charge.

Bottomless Soup & Salad – Unlimited refills. Chose any of our delicious soups and a House Salad. Served with warm tostado chips and salsa.

Sandwiches & Handhelds:

Served with home-style fries. On all sandwiches I ask the waitperson to substitute a vegetable or a small salad for the home-style fries.

Grilled Chicken Sandwich – Chicken breast with Applewood smoked bacon, fresh sliced tomato, lettuce, Swiss cheese, & honey-mustard. I ask the waitperson to ask the chef to substitute extra tomato for the bacon.

Buffalo Chicken Ranch Sandwich – Crispy chicken with our spicy buffalo sauce, fresh sliced tomato, lettuce, and house-made ranch. I ask the waitperson to ask the chef to substitute grilled chicken for the crispy chicken.

Classic Turkey Toasted Sandwich – Thinly sliced turkey with lettuce, fresh sliced tomato, provolone cheese & mayo on wheat Texas toast.

Craft Burgers:

New savory burgers crafted to perfection, with fresh ingredients. Served with new house-made garlic dill pickles & home-style fries. Now more ways to make it your own – Substitute new patties on request: 2 thin beef patties or turkey patty. On all burgers I ask the waitperson to substitute a vegetable or a small salad for the home-style fries.

Classic Bacon Burger – Topped with Applewood smoked bacon, melted sharp cheddar cheese, new house-made garlic dill pickles, fresh leaf lettuce, tomato, sliced red onion and new Chili's signature sauce. I ask the waitperson to ask the chef to substitute extra tomato for the bacon.

Oldtimer® With Cheese – Chili's classic – improved! Hand seasoned beef patty, seared to perfection. Topped with new house-made garlic dill pickles, fresh leaf lettuce, tomato, sliced red onions & mustard.

Oldtimer® – Chili's classic – improved! Hand seasoned beef patty, seared to perfection. Topped with new house-made garlic dill pickles, fresh leaf lettuce, tomato, sliced red onions & mustard.

Lighter Choices:

Mango-Chile Chicken – Grilled chicken with 6 pepper blend, drizzled with spicy habanero mango glaze & topped with chopped mango, cilantro, house-made pico de gallo & fresh diced avocado. Served with rice and steamed broccoli. I ask the waitperson to ask the chef to substitute extra broccoli for the rice and the avocado.

Grilled Chicken Salad – Grilled chicken served over fresh field greens, topped with diced tomatoes, house-made corn and black bean salsa, 3 cheese blend and honey-lime vinaigrette.

Lighter Choice 6 oz. Sirloin – 100% Choice USDA sirloin grilled to order with carne asada rub featuring red chilies, garlic and pepper. Topped with house-made pico de gallo and served with steamed broccoli.

Fresh Mex:

Your classic favorites – plus some fresh new surprises!

Mix & Match Fajitas – We're reinvented our classic favorite! Our signature sizzling fajitas served with sliced bell peppers & caramelized onions, topped with chipotle-garlic butter and chopped cilantro. Served with warm flour or corn tortillas & fresh new toppings. Choose from grilled chicken or steak or both.

Make It A Combo:

Why settle for one entrée when you can have the taste of two? Choose any two, all served with loaded mashed potatoes &

steamed broccoli. I ask the waitperson to ask the chef to substitute extra steamed broccoli for the mashed potatoes.

Monterey Chicken®

Margareta Grilled Chicken – Lighter choice item.

6 oz. Classic Sirloin – Also available as a lighter choice item.

Ribs & Steaks:

Enjoy the fall-off-the-bone goodness of our world-famous baby back ribs slow smoked over pecan wood. Choose from Original BBQ Sauce or Memphis Dry Rub. (Notice: Approximate pre-cooked weights, actual weight may vary. May be cooked to order.)

Classic Ribeye – 100% USDA thick-cut steak marbled for maximum flavor & topped with garlic butter. Served with loaded mashed potatoes & steamed broccoli. I ask the waitperson to ask the chef to substitute extra broccoli for mashed potatoes.

Classic Sirloin – 10 oz. 100% USDA Choice 10 oz. sirloin with Chili's seasoning & topped with garlic butter. Served with loaded mashed potatoes & steamed broccoli. Plus up your steak with sautéed mushrooms for an additional charge. I ask the waitperson to ask the chef to substitute extra broccoli for the mashed potatoes.

Classic Sirloin – 6 oz. 100% USDA Choice 10 oz. sirloin with Chili's seasoning & topped with garlic butter. Served with loaded mashed potatoes & steamed broccoli. Plus up your steak with sautéed mushrooms for an additional charge. I ask the waitperson to ask the chef to substitute extra broccoli for the mashed potatoes.

Desserts:

Skillet Toffee Fudge Brownie – Oven-baked toffee brownie topped with vanilla ice cream, drizzled with caramel sauce &

topped with toffee pieces. (†This dish contains nuts.)

<u>Molten Chocolate Cake</u> – Indulge in moist chocolate cake with a melted chocolate center topped with vanilla ice cream & a thin chocolate shell.

Claim Jumper
Chain Restaurant

Appetizers:

<u>Spinach Artichoke Dip</u> – Blended with aged Parmesan and slow baked. Served with tortilla chips.

<u>Tomato Bruschetta</u> – Tomato, basil and balsamic relish garnished with shredded Parmesan and served with grilled tomato herbed bread.

<u>Buffalo Chicken Bites</u> – Tossed in our signature buffalo sauce and served with celery, carrots and ranch dressing for dipping. I ask the waitperson to ask the chef to leave off the breading.

<u>Sliders</u> – Mini burgers topped with double thick Cheddar. Ask your server for "The Works". BBQ chicken also available.

Homemade Soups:

Made-from-scratch daily.

<u>Vegetable Soup</u> – Potatoes, carrots, celery, green beans, red peppers and corn fresh from the garden served in vegetable stock. Served with a dollop of basil and walnut pesto.

<u>Creamy Chicken Tortilla</u> – A blend of rotisserie chicken, chilies and onions, topped with homemade tortilla strips. I ask the waitperson to ask the chef to leave off the tortilla strips.

Garden Fresh Salads:

<u>House Salad</u> – Tomatoes, mushrooms carrots, Cheddar cheese, diced egg, crisp bacon and croutons. I ask the waitperson to ask the chef to substitute extra tomatoes and mushrooms for the bacon and croutons.

<u>Spinach Salad</u> – Tossed with crunchy noodles, diced red onions, tomatoes, Mandarin oranges, dried cranberries, feta

cheese, glazed pecans, sesame seeds and our homemade balsamic vinaigrette dressing. I ask the waitperson to ask the chef to substitute extra tomatoes for the crunchy noodles.

Chinese Chicken Salad – Char-grilled chicken with crunchy noodles, almonds, sesame seeds, green onions, carrots and cilantro, tossed with a sweet and spicy peanut dressing. I ask the waitperson to ask the chef to substitute extra carrots for the crunchy noodles.

California Citrus Chicken Salad – Char-grilled chicken with Mandarin oranges, green apples, avocado, dried cranberries, red onions, glazed pecans, bleu cheese crumbles and green onions. Tossed with our signature citrus vinaigrette dressing. I ask the waitperson to ask the chef to substitute extra green apples for the avocado.

Chicken Caesar Salad – Char-grilled or blackened chicken, crisp Romaine tossed with aged Parmesan, croutons and creamy Caesar dressing. I order the char-grilled chicken and ask the waitperson to ask the chef to substitute extra Romaine for the croutons and to substitute bleu cheese dressing for the Caesar dressing.

Chopped Cobb Salad – Char-grilled chicken, bleu cheese crumbles, avocado, bacon, diced egg and tomatoes with homemade bleu cheese dressing. For an additional charge can substitute Char-grilled beef tenderloin. I ask the waitperson to ask the chef to substitute extra tomatoes for the avocado and bacon.

Hill Country Salad – Chunks of lightly fried chicken and grated Cheddar cheese on a bed of crisp greens with tomatoes, bacon, eggs and croutons tossed with ranch or honey mustard dressing. I ask the waitperson to ask the chef to substitute char-grilled chicken for the fried chicken and to substitute extra crisp greens for the bacon and croutons.

Produce Bar – Create your own salad from an array of fresh

ingredients. Produce bar and a bowl of soup.

California Citrus Salad – Mandarin oranges, green apples, avocado, dried cranberries, red onion, glazed pecans, bleu cheese crumbles and green onion. Tossed with mixed greens and our signature citrus vinaigrette dressing. I ask the waitperson to ask the chef to substitute extra mixed greens for the avocado.

Favorites:

Served with a small green salad or small Caesar salad or a cup of soup. I order the small green salad.

Tenderloin Tips – Grilled tenderloin tips tossed in an herb demi-glace with sautéed mushrooms and grilled onions atop mashed potatoes. Served with roasted vegetables. I ask the waitperson to ask the chef to substitute extra roasted vegetables for the mashed potatoes.

Hickory Chicken – Marinated and grilled boneless chicken breast with our smoky BBQ sauce then topped with sautéed mushrooms and topped with melted Jack cheese. Served with mashed potatoes and green beans. I ask the waitperson to ask the chef to substitute extra green beans for the mashed potatoes.

Simply Grilled Chicken Breast – Marinated, grilled and served with mashed potatoes and roasted vegetables. I ask the waitperson to ask the chef to substitute green beans for the mashed potatoes.

Burgers & Sandwiches:

Served with fresh greens and tomato and choice of one: Spicy Peanut Thai Slaw, Fresh-Cut Fruit, Seasoned French Fries. All burgers are cooked medium well unless otherwise requested. I order the Spicy Peanut Thai Slaw.

Hickory BBQ Burger – Brushed with mesquite BBQ sauce, topped with smoked bacon, smoked Gouda and Thousand Island dressing. I ask the waitperson to ask the chef to leave off the bacon and Thousand Island dressing.

Classic Cheeseburger – Double-thick Cheddar and Thousand Island dressing. I ask the waitperson to ask the chef to substitute Dijon mustard for the Thousand Island dressing.

Sliders – Mini burgers topped with double-thick Cheddar. Ask your server for "The Works". BBQ chicken also available.

Roast Turkey on Wheatberry – With tomato, crisp greens and mayo.

Portabella Sandwich – Layers of portabella mushroom, balsamic dressed spinach, roasted red pepper, avocado and goat cheese, served on baked tomato herb bread spread with Dijon mustard and basil walnut pesto. I ask the waitperson to ask the chef to substitute extra spinach for the avocado.

Original Tri-Tip Dip – Slow roasted and simmered in French onion broth with caramelized onions, roasted pasilla peppers and smoked Gouda on a French roll with au jus or sweet BBQ sauce. I order the au jus.

Cashew Chicken Salad Sandwich – Diced with cashews, celery, and curried aioli on fresh baked tomato herb bread.

BBQ Chicken Sandwich – Julienned and tossed with sweet BBQ sauce, smoked Gouda and mayo on fresh baked tomato herb bread.

Grilled Steaks:

All steaks are aged, seasoned and flame-broiled, then finished with garlic-herb butter. All grilled steaks are served with a small green salad or small Caesar salad or a cup of soup and one side. I order the small green salad.

Meritage Smothered Steak – 8 oz. sirloin smothered with

grilled onions, sautéed mushrooms and a red wine demi-glace.

Sesame Glazed Smothered Steak – 8 oz. sirloin smothered with roasted vegetables and a sweet Asian sauce, topped with wontons and chives. I ask the waitperson to ask the chef to leave off the wontons.

High Sierra Smothered Steak – 8 oz. sirloin smothered with roasted pasilla peppers, grilled onions, bleu cheese butter and chives.

Top Sirloin – Certified Angus Beef® top sirloin. Served with a side of red wine demi-glace. 7oz. or 9oz.

Porterhouse Steak – Two steaks in one! Our famous 20 oz. USDA Choice bone-in NY strip and filet.

Filet Mignon – 7 oz. center-cut filet served with a side of red wine demi-glace.

Ribeye Steak – 12 oz. hand-cut, boneless USDA Choice.

Bone-in-Ribeye Steak – 24 oz. Certified Angus Beef® bone-in Ribeye is our most flavorful steak.

New York Strip – 12 oz. center-cut USDA Choice.

Sides:

Green Beans

Roasted Vegetables

Cheese Broccoli

Great Steak Additions:

Sautéed mushrooms or bleu cheese butter.

Steak Toppings:

Asian Vegetable

Bleu Cheese with Peppers & Onions

Red Wine with Mushrooms & Onions

Original Rotisserie Specialties And Combos:

Original rotisserie specialties and combos are served with roasted vegetables and one side and a small green salad, small Caesar salad or a cup of soup. I order the small green salad.

Rotisserie Chicken – Our original recipe since 1977. A half chicken seasoned, slow cooked over open flames and roasted to perfection.

Roasted Tri-Tip – Certified Angus Beef ® slow roasted and sliced over herb demi-glace. Served only medium rare to medium.

Roasted Tri-Tip & Chicken – Certified Angus Beef ® slow-roasted and sliced over herb demi-glace pared with rotisserie chicken.

Pastas:

Served with a small green salad or a small Caesar salad or a cup of soup.

Absolute Tortellini – Cheese tortellini and blackened chicken, tossed in a vodka tomato cream sauce with bacon and topped with shredded Parmesan and fresh parsley. I ask the waitperson to ask the chef to prepare my pasta without bacon.

Black Tie Chicken Pasta – Blackened chicken, bow tie pasta, spinach tortellini and oven-roasted tomatoes, tossed in creamy Alfredo sauce.

Chicken & Broccoli Alfredo – Grilled chicken, fresh broccoli and egg noodles, tossed in creamy Alfredo sauce.

Portabella Pasta – Grilled portabella mushrooms, roasted red bell peppers and fresh spinach, sautéed in a sherry Parmesan cream sauce tossed in fettuccine and topped with crumbled goat cheese.

Pesto Primavera – Farfalle and cheese tortellini, tossed in our basil walnut pesto, topped with roasted carrots, squash, zucchini, red onion, broccoli, artichoke hearts and roasted tomatoes, topped with Parmesan cheese.

Homemade Desserts:

Original Scratch Carrot Cake – Three layers of subtly spiced carrot cake, generously covered with cream cheese frosting.

Brownie Finale – Double chocolate walnut brownie served warm and topped with fudge frosting, vanilla ice cream, whipped cream and toasted almonds.

Italian Lemon Cake – Five layers of rich cream cake, filled and topped with white chocolate lemon filling.

Lunch Menu:

Soups, Salads & Sandwiches.

See menu above.

CJ Favorites:

See Favorites above.

Cooper's Hawk Winery & Restaurants
Chain Restaurant

Appetizers:

Thai Lettuce Wraps – Soy glazed chicken, julienne of vegetables, crunchy wontons, Bibb lettuce with peanut, cashew, and soy caramel sauces. I ask the waitperson to ask the chef to leave off the wontons.

Chicken Al Pastor Stuffed with Mushrooms – Traditional Mexican spices, chicken, chorizo, pepperjack cheese, cilantro, crispy tortilla strips, sour cream, chipotle tomato sauce. I ask the waitperson to ask the chef to leave off the tortilla strips and substitute extra cheese for the chorizo.

Chef Matt's Cheese Platter – Artisan cheeses for the novice as well as the cheese enthusiast. Served with lavash crisps. I ask the waitperson to ask the chef to leave off the lavash crisps.

Appetizer Salads:

Plain Ol' House – Cucumbers, carrots, croutons, tomatoes, and dressing on the side. I ask the waitperson to ask the chef to substitute extra tomatoes for the cucumbers and croutons.

Caesar Pesto – Romaine, herb-roasted croutons, creamy Caesar pesto dressing, shaved Asiago, parmesan lavash. I ask the waitperson to ask the chef to substitute extra romaine for the croutons and lavash and to substitute blue cheese dressing for the Caesar dressing.

Chopped Wedge – Red onion, sweet grape tomatoes, Applewood smoked bacon, red wine herb vinaigrette, blue cheese dressing. I ask the waitperson to ask the chef to substitute extra tomatoes for the bacon.

Flatbreads:

Caprese – Ripe tomatoes, mozzarella, red onion, pesto, julienne basil, and balsamic glaze.

Roasted Vegetable & Goat Cheese – Mozzarella, roasted grape tomatoes, pesto, julienne basil, and balsamic glaze.

Carne Asada – Sliced skirt steak, pesto, mozzarella, roasted chili sauce, and cilantro.

Chopped Salads:

Mediterranean – Cucumbers, red onion, asparagus, Kalamata olives, mild Giardiniera, sweet grape tomatoes, feta cheese, red wine and lemon herb vinaigrette. Can add chicken for an additional charge. I ask the waitperson to ask the chef to substitute extra grape tomatoes for the cucumbers.

Blackened Bleu Steak – Sliced skirt steak, onions, tomatoes, crispy onion strings, Italian vinaigrette, and bleu cheese dressing. I ask the waitperson to ask the chef to substitute extra tomatoes for the crispy onion strings.

Napa Chicken – Apples, goat cheese, dried cherries, corn, avocado, toasted almonds, cilantro, tomatoes, chicken, and honey mustard vinaigrette. I ask the waitperson to ask the chef to substitute extra apples for the corn and avocado.

Soups:

Tortilla Soup – I ask the waitperson to ask the chef to leave off the tortilla strips.

Artisan Soup of the Day – Ask your server for today's selection.

Burgers & Sandwiches:

Served with your choice of seasoned fries, fresh fruit or Asian slaw. I order the Asian slaw. Any beef patty may be substituted with a turkey patty.

Classic Cheeseburger – Lettuce, tomato, choice of cheese, seasoned mayo, crispy onion strings. I ask the waitperson to ask the chef to substitute extra tomato for the crispy onion strings.

Bleu Cheese & Crispy Onion Burger – Melted bleu cheese, crispy onion strings, lettuce, tomato, and chipotle mayo. I ask the waitperson to ask the chef to substitute extra tomato for the crispy onion strings.

Jalapeno Bacon Burger – Pepperjack cheese, crispy onion strings, lettuce, tomato, and chipotle mayo. I ask the waitperson to ask the chef to substitute extra pepperjack cheese for the jalapeno bacon and crispy onion strings.

Turkey Burger – Fresh ground all-natural turkey, herbs, lemon, seasoned mayo, lettuce, and tomato.

The Prime – Slow-roasted prime rib, seasoned mayo, and house made steak jus.

Mediterranean Vegetable Sandwich – Grilled vegetables, organic greens, hummus, cucumber and herb-feta cream. I ask the waitperson to ask the chef to substitute extra organic greens for the cucumber.

Southwest Chicken Sandwich – Lettuce, pico de gallo, guacamole, pepperjack cheese, chipotle mayo and jalapeno bacon. I ask the waitperson to ask the chef to substitute extra pepperjack cheese for the guacamole and jalapeno bacon.

Cilantro Ranch Chicken Sandwich – Cheddar, Applewood smoked bacon, avocado, cilantro ranch, seasoned mayo. I ask the waitperson to ask the chef to substitute tomatoes for the bacon and avocado.

Crispy Parmesan Chicken Sandwich – Marinara, mild Giardiniera, Provolone, and pesto mayo. I ask the waitperson to ask the chef to leave the breading off the chicken and to grill it or sauté it.

Honey-Smoked Turkey & Brie – Thin-sliced red apple, honey mustard mayo, candied walnuts.

Lunch Sized Entrees:

See chicken selection below.

Chicken:

Anne's Chicken Saltimbocca – Prosciutto, Provolone, garlic, sage, artichoke hearts, capers, tomatoes, white wine lemon sauce, Mary's potatoes, and asparagus. I ask the waitperson to ask the chef to leave off the prosciutto and to substitute extra asparagus for the potatoes.

Dana's Parmesan-Crusted Chicken – Garlic green beans, tomato basil relish, lemon butter, and Betty's potatoes. I ask the waitperson to ask the chef to substitute extra green beans for the potatoes.

Cooper's Hawk Chicken Giardiniera – Parmesan breaded chicken, mild Giardiniera, shaved parmesan, and Mary's potatoes. I ask the waitperson to ask the chef to prepare the chicken without breading and to substitute green beans for the potatoes.

Chicken Madeira- Mushrooms, Provolone, Mary's potatoes, and asparagus. I ask the waitperson to ask the chef to substitute extra asparagus for the potatoes.

Ellie's Chicken Piccata – Lemon butter, caper sauce, angel hair pasta. I ask the waitperson to ask the chef to substitute roasted vegetables for the pasta.

Pork & Beef:

Trio of Medallions – Horseradish, bleu cheese, and parmesan-crusted filet medallions, Mary's potatoes, and asparagus. I ask the waitperson to ask the chef to substitute green beans for the potatoes.

Churrasco Grilled Steak – Chimichurri rubbed skirt steak, parmesan fries, roasted vegetables, and cilantro-lime aioli. I ask the waitperson to ask the chef to substitute extra roasted vegetables for the potatoes.

Filet Mignon – Herbed butter, crispy onion strings, broccoli florets, choice of side. I order roasted vegetables for the side and ask the waitperson to ask the chef to substitute extra broccoli for the onion strings.

New York Strip – Roasted vegetables and choice of a side. I order green beans.

Signature Crusts & Toppings:

Bleu Cheese

Horseradish

Parmesan Crust

Sherry Glazed Mushrooms

Signature Sides:

Asian Slaw

Roasted Vegetables

Pasta:

Angel Hair Napolitano – Fresh garlic, chili flakes, chicken, broccoli, San Maranzo tomato sauce, extra virgin olive oil.

Chicken Linguini Reggiano – Sweet grape tomatoes, Portobello mushrooms, spinach, and garlic cream.

House Made Desserts:

Crumbled Apple Pie – Warm caramel sauce and vanilla bean ice cream.

Chocolate Pretzel Bread Pudding – Whipped cream, toasted white chocolate, rum caramel and vanilla sauce.

Classic Crème Brulee

Banana Caramel Ice Cream Sandwich – Caramelized bananas, banana bread, warm buttered rum caramel sauce, and vanilla bean ice cream.

Truffles & Chocolate Covered Strawberries:

I eat the dark chocolate.

Chocolate-Covered Strawberry

Chocolate Truffle

Dressel's Public House
St. Louis, MO

Lunch:

Snacks:

House Marinated Roasted Olives – Gordal, Picholine, and Cuquillo

Soups and Salads:

French Onion Soup – Three cheese blend and croutons. I ask the waitperson to ask the chef to prepare my onion soup without croutons.

Stockpot Special of the Day

Candy Apple Salad – Mixed greens, apple, blue cheese, candied peanuts, cider-tarragon vinaigrette.

Romaine Wedge Salad – Bacon, pickled red onion, 8 minute egg, cornbread croutons, and parmesan peppercorn dressing. I ask the waitperson to ask the chef to substitute extra lettuce for the bacon and the croutons.

Public Plates:

Three Cheese Board – Chef's selection, fresh & dried fruits, nuts, house-made jams & chutneys.

Sandwiches:

Served with mixed greens.

Dressel's Burger – Ridgley Farms Missouri beef, aged cheddar, onion jam, and brioche bun.

Lamb Burger – Apricot chutney, chevre, house bread & butter pickles, and brioche bun.

Grilled Chicken Sandwich – Candied bacon, apple fennel slaw, blue cheese aioli, lettuce, and ciabatta bun.

Dinner:

See menu above.

Plates:

Beer Brined Chicken – Pan seared breast, everything spatzle, apple cider sauerkraut, wild mushroom jus. I ask the waitperson to ask the chef to substitute a vegetable for the spatzle.

Ridgley Beef – buckwheat Taranga polenta, pickled Italian heirloom pepper relish, gorgonzola, and fresh picked herbs. I ask the waitperson to ask the chef to substitute a vegetable for the polenta.

Elephant Bar
Global Grill/Wok Kitchen
Chain Restaurant

Openers:

Our Openers are a variety of bold global flavors perfect to be shared with family and friends or to mix and match to create your own unique dining adventure.

Korean Beef Tacos – Marinated beef sirloin with cabbage, carrots, tomatoes, cilantro, avocado and sour cream. Served with Asian slaw and roasted tomato salsa. I ask the waitperson to ask the chef to substitute extra tomatoes for the avocado.

Wok-Fired Chicken Lettuce Wraps – Chopped chicken, water chestnuts, toasted coconut flakes and roasted cashews with fresh Vera Cruz salsa, marinated cucumbers and crispy chilled lettuce leaves. Served with our tamarind macadamia nut sauce. I ask the waitperson to ask the chef to substitute extra water chestnuts for the cucumbers.

Parmesan Crusted Green Beans – Fresh green beans quick-fried in a crispy parmesan crust and served with a sweet chili sauce.

Warm and Spicy Artichoke Dip – Blend of artichoke hearts, cheese, fresh spinach and spices. Served with corn tortilla chips. I do not eat the tortilla chips.

Side Salads + Soups:

Fresh Pear and Gorgonzola – Served over Bibb lettuce, arugula and watercress. Tossed in walnut cider vinaigrette with glazed walnuts.

Crisp Iceberg Wedge – Refreshing crisp wedge of iceberg lettuce with 1000 Island or blue cheese dressing, crisp bacon, diced tomatoes and chopped eggs. I order the blue cheese dressing. I ask the waitperson to ask the chef to substitute extra tomatoes for the bacon.

Citrus Side Salad – Mix of chopped iceberg, green leaf and romaine lettuce with carrots and red cabbage. Tossed with avocado, green apples, caramelized walnuts, green onions, gorgonzola cheese crumbles, dried cranberries and mandarin oranges. Finished with our tropical honey citrus dressing. I ask the waitperson to ask the chef to substitute extra green apples for the avocado.

Certified Organic Field Greens – Mix of farmer's seasonal selection. Tossed in balsamic mustard dressing with crumbled gorgonzola cheese and caramelized walnuts.

Tomato Basil Bisque

French Onion Soup

Soup of the Day

Entrée Salads:

Market Cobb Salad – Wood-fired shredded BBQ chicken breast, hickory-smoked bacon, avocado, tomato, mushrooms, crumbled gorgonzola cheese and chopped eggs over crisp chopped mixed greens. Choice of balsamic mustard, blue cheese or ranch dressing. I order the balsamic mustard or the blue cheese dressing. I ask the waitperson to ask the chef to substitute extra tomatoes and mushrooms for the bacon and avocado.

Thai-High Sweet and Zesty Chicken Salad – Wok-seared chicken tossed in a ginger-spiced sweet and sour dressing. Served over mixed greens with carrots diced tomatoes, cucumbers and wonton strips. I ask the waitperson to ask the chef to substitute extra greens for the cucumbers and wonton strips.

<u>Citrus Salad with Grilled Chicken</u> – Lemon herb wood-fired chicken breast over a fresh mix of greens with carrots and red cabbage. Tossed with avocado, caramelized walnuts, mandarin oranges, green apples, dried cranberries, gorgonzola cheese crumbles and green onions. Finished with tropical honey citrus dressing. I ask the waitperson to ask the chef to substitute extra green apples for the avocado.

<u>California Fruit Salad</u> – Organic lettuce tossed with mixed fruit, tropical honey citrus dressing and orange blossom drizzle, topped with fresh mint. Chicken can be added for an extra charge. I ask the waitperson to ask the chef to leave off the fresh mint.

Salad Dressings:

Our side salads use 1 oz. of dressing and our entrée salads use 2-3 oz.

<u>Red Ginger Vinaigrette</u>

<u>Tropical Honey Citrus</u>

<u>Walnut Cider Vinaigrette</u>

<u>Citrus Dijon Herb</u>

<u>Balsamic Mustard</u>

<u>Bleu Cheese</u>

Build Your Own Burger:

<u>Step 1: Chose a Protein</u> – 1/2 Ground beef patty or chicken breast.

<u>Step 2: Chose a Bun</u> – Egg bun or focaccia bread.

<u>Step 3: Cheese</u> – Cheddar, Swiss, Provolone, Monterey Jack, or gorgonzola crumbles.

<u>Step 4: Premium Sauces</u> – I do not use them. I use mustard.

<u>Step 5:</u> – Included on all burgers – lettuce, tomatoes, pickles, and

onions (raw or sautéed). More toppings: Sautéed mushrooms for an additional charge.

Step 6: Chose a Side – Coleslaw or garden salad.

Sandwiches:

Each sandwich is served with a choice of one of the following sides: Garden Salad or Coleslaw.

The Smokehouse – Skinless chicken breast basted with our own BBQ sauce with smoked bacon, ham, melted cheddar cheese and crisp onion strings. I ask the waitperson to ask the chef to substitute lettuce, tomatoes and pickles for the bacon, ham, and onion strings.

Sirloin Steak Sandwich – Tender 8 oz. (pre-cooked weight) sirloin steak fire-grilled over oak wood, topped with our flavorful steak butter and crispy onion straws. Served open-faced on toasted parmesan garlic bread slice with a side of fresh fruit. I ask the waitperson to ask the chef to substitute either grilled or raw onion for the onion straws.

Philly Cheese Steak – Thinly sliced ribeye steak grilled with onions, mushrooms and sweet peppers. Finished with Provolone stacked high on a toasted French roll.

Classic French Dip – Seasoned roast beef, sliced and piled high on a grilled French roll. Served with au jus. Cheese can be added for an additional charge.

Wood-Fired Grill:

Our steaks are all USDA Choice and aged a minimum of 21 days. We serve only fresh chicken. Add a small garden salad for an additional charge.

Ribeye and Sautéed Chicken Marsala – A 12 oz. (pre-cooked weight) wood-fired Ribeye topped with our flavorful steak butter paired with two chicken medallions, sautéed with fresh mushrooms and our Marsala wine sauce. Served with garlic mashed potatoes and fresh vegetables. I ask the waitperson to ask the chef to substitute extra fresh vegetables for the potatoes.

Top Sirloin – An 8 oz. (pre-cooked weight) wood-fired center cut sirloin topped with our flavorful steak butter and served with fresh vegetables and garlic mashed potatoes. I ask the waitperson to ask the chef to substitute extra fresh vegetables for the potatoes.

Lemon Garlic Chicken Breast – Wood-fired lemon garlic chicken breast topped with oven-roasted tomatoes and basil pesto. Served with a fresh blend of steamed vegetables, brown rice and grilled lemon. I ask the waitperson to ask the chef to substitute extra steamed vegetables for the rice.

Wok-Fired Specialties:

Our chicken is fresh. All vegetables in our wok dishes are farm fresh. All wok-fired specialties are served with steamed white or brown rice. Add a garden salad for an additional charge. On all wok-fired specialties I ask the waitperson to ask the chef to substitute fresh or steamed vegetables for the rice.

Mongolian Beef – Thinly sliced, quick-seared sirloin with shitake mushrooms, jupons hot chili peppers and green onions, tossed in soy-ginger-garlic spiced sauce. Served over fresh vegetables.

Crispy Teriyaki Chicken – Wok-fired teriyaki-glazed chicken served with fresh vegetables, all tossed in a mushroom soy-ginger-garlic sauce. Finished with green onions and toasted sesame seeds. I ask the waitperson to ask the chef to leave the breading off the chicken.

Orange Chicken – Lightly battered and quick-fried chicken, wok-fired with fresh vegetables tossed in our signature orange sauce. I ask the waitperson to ask the chef to leave the batter off the chicken.

Thai-High Chicken Stir-Fry – We've taken our signature salad and made it a wok-fired dish. Chicken with fresh vegetables tossed in our ginger-spiced sweet sauce and sour dressing.

Global Specialties:

We serve only fresh chicken. A garden salad can be added for an additional charge.

Braised Lamb Shanks – Two large, fork tender New Zealand lamb shanks in a sauce of roasted garlic, tomatoes and rosemary. Served with garlic mashed potatoes and sautéed vegetables. I ask the waitperson to ask the chef to substitute extra sautéed vegetables for the potatoes.

Parmesan Chicken and Tuscan Style Shrimp – Parmesan crusted chicken paired with shrimp. Parmesan crusted chicken available without the shrimp. I order it without the shrimp.

Sautéed Chicken Marsala – Three Chicken medallions with sautéed mushrooms in a Marsala wine sauce. Served with garlic mashed potatoes and sautéed spinach. Topped with Parmesan cheese. I ask the waitperson to ask the chef to substitute sautéed vegetables for the mashed potatoes.

Lunch Specialties:

Smaller portions of dinner entrees. See listing above.

Farina Alto
Pizzeria & Wine Bar
Albuquerque, NM

Antipasti:

Oven Roasted Assorted Italian Olives

Meatballs Al Forno Balsamico

Antipasto Platter – Roasted artichoke hearts, cured meats, imported cheeses, olives, fresh mozzarella, Calabrese peppers, pepperoncini, tomato, and roasted red peppers. I ask the waitperson to ask the chef to substitute extra imported cheeses for the cured meats.

Sautéed Mushrooms

Insalata:

Caprese Salad – House mozzarella, fresh tomato, basil, evoo.

Verde Salad – Organic lettuces, roasted walnuts, apples, oregonzola, Champaign vinaigrette.

Baby Spinach Salad – Sliced mushrooms, shallots, house pancetta, chopped egg, balsamic vinaigrette. I ask the waitperson to ask the chef to substitute extra spinach for the pancetta.

Chopped Vegetable Salad – (to share), red wine vinaigrette.

Grilled Chicken Breast Salad – Arugula, roasted red pepper, house mozzarella, tomato, capers, olives, balsamic vinaigrette.

Entrees:

Meatball Calzone – Marinara, mozzarella, ricotta, spinach and garlic.

Semolina Spaghetti – Meatballs and tomato sauce.

Chicken Piccata – Chicken scaloppini, roasted Rosemary potatoes, seasonal vegetables and lemon caper sauce. I ask the waitperson to ask the chef to substitute extra seasonal vegetables for the potatoes.

Pizza:

Margherita – Tomato sauce, house mozzarella and fresh basil.

Melanzane – Marinara, mozzarella, eggplant, basil and oregano.

Funghi – Mozzarella, fontina, taleggio, mushrooms, shallot and thyme.

Bianca – Mozzarella, ricotta, artichoke hearts, sage and truffle oil.

Meatball – Marinara, mozzarella, ricotta, meatballs, spinach and garlic.

Flamez
Albuquerque, NM

Burger Saladz:

Lebanese (Fatoush) – Romaine lettuce, cucumber, tomatoes, peppers, scallions, radishes, pita chips and lemon-sumac vinaigrette served with a beef Shawerma. I ask the waitperson to ask the chef to substitute extra lettuce and tomatoes for the cucumber and pita chips.

Greek – Lettuce, tomatoes, cucumbers, red onion, Kalamata olives, feta cheese & a Colorado lamb burger. I ask the waitperson to ask the chef to substitute extra red onion for the cucumbers.

Chopped Salad – Lettuce, bacon tomatoes, onions, peppers, cucumber, cheddar cheese & grilled steak burger. I ask the waitperson to ask the chef to substitute extra peppers and onions for the bacon and cucumber.

Wedge Salad – Romaine wedge, tomatoes, bacon, bleu cheese & grilled steak burger. I ask the waitperson to ask the chef to substitute red onion for the bacon.

Caesar – Romaine lettuce, parmesan cheese, garlic croutons & grilled chicken. I ask the waitperson to ask the chef to substitute extra romaine for the croutons and to substitute bleu cheese dressing for the Caesar dressing.

Burger Bowlz:

All burger bowls are served with a grilled 8 oz. hamburger steak.

All American – Mashed potatoes, sautéed mushrooms, caramelized onions, & cheddar cheese. I ask the waitperson to ask the chef to substitute extra mushrooms for the mashed potatoes.

Asian – Steamed rice, onions, peppers, scallions, mushrooms & soy ginger sauce. I ask the waitperson to ask the chef to substitute extra peppers for the rice.

Italian – Asparagus and mushroom risotto, & parmesan cheese.

Russian Bowl (Stroganoff) – Egg noodles, mushrooms, & tangy pickles in a rich, classic stroganoff sauce.

Choose A Burger:

All burgers are served with tomato, onion, lettuce, pickle & choice of cheese.

Black Angus Beef

Grass Fed Beef

American Buffalo

Venison

Colorado Lamb

All White Turkey

Choose A Cheese:

Swiss

Monterey Jack

Cheddar

Provolone

Choose A Side:

Personal Green Salad

Grilled Vegetables

Extra Dressing

Toppingz:

Green Chile

Sautéed Mushrooms

Caramelized Onions

Sandwiches & Wraps from Around the World:

All sandwiches are served with a personal green salad.

Chicken Club – Grilled chicken breast, mayo, bacon, lettuce, tomato & Jack cheese. I ask the waitperson to ask the chef to substitute extra tomato for the bacon and to leave off the center slice of bread.

Caprese – Fresh mozzarella, tomatoes, arugula, fresh basil & balsamic vinaigrette.

Gyro – Spiced grilled lamb, tomatoes, lettuce, feta cheese & Greek yogurt sauce.

Smoked Turkey Breast – Smoked turkey breast, cranberry mayo, caramelized onions, bacon & brie cheese. I ask the waitperson to ask the chef to substitute extra caramelized onions for the bacon.

Falafel – Chickpea fritters, onion, tomatoes, sumac & garlicky tahina sauce.

Torta De Carne Asada – Grilled, marinated skirt steak, onions, peppers, Jack cheese, cilantro & smoked jalapeno mayo.

Shawerma – Onion, tomatoes, lettuce, sumac & garlicky tahina sauce. Choose chicken or beef.

Dessertz:

Ice Cream – Chocolate, vanilla bean or butter pecan.

Carrot Bread Pudding – Carrot bread pudding, butter pecan ice cream & cardamom caramel sauce.

<u>Apple Torte</u> – Granny Smith apples, cranberries, walnuts & salted caramel sauce.

<u>Mango Cheesecake</u>

Giovanni's Kitchen
Ladue, MO

Salads:

Our Caesar – Romaine hearts, rapini and fresh kale, sundried tomatoes and focaccia croutons tossed with homemade Caesar dressing and Pecorino Romano. I ask the waitperson to ask the chef to leave off the croutons and to substitute balsamic vinegar for the Caesar dressing.

Burrata Al Pomodoro – Fresh, creamy Mozzarella, olive oil and a hint of balsamic vinegar, sliced tomatoes and basil, served on a bed of mixed greens.

Rucolina E Spinaci – Arugula, baby spoon spinach and crispy guanciale tossed with homemade red wine vinaigrette, Caciocavallo cheese and fresh grapes. I ask the waitperson to ask the chef to substitute extra spinach for the grapes.

Novella – Tender Bibb lettuce tossed in a light vinaigrette, honey, Gorgonzola crumbles, Mozzarella and grilled focaccia. I ask the waitperson to ask the chef to leave off the grilled focaccia.

Soups:

Minestrone

Italian Egg Drop

Pizzette & Flatbreads:

Classic Margherita Pizzette

Portobello and Fontina Flatbread

Artisan Pasta:

Bucatini All' Amatricana – Hollow spaghetti, guanciale in

lightly spiced San Maranzo tomato sauce sautéed with Pecorino Romano, basil and extra virgin olive oil.

Tortellacci Alla Fonduta – Large tortellini, filled with Fontina, Ricotta, Parmigiano and Asiago. Served in a light tomato basil sauce.

Mezzemaniche Alla Puttanesca – Olives, garlic and capers in a spicy San Maranzo tomato sauce and large rigatoni pasta tossed with Parmigiano Reggiano.

Entrée:

All entrees are served with mashed potatoes. I ask the waitperson to ask the chef to substitute sautéed spinach for the potatoes.

Parmigiana Di Pollo – Tender chicken breast, breaded and pan fried. Served with fresh "pomodorina" sauce, homemade Mozzarella, basil and a dusting of Parmigiano. I ask the waitperson to ask the chef to prepare the chicken breast without breading.

Rotolini Di Polo – Free range chicken breast rolled and stuffed with imported Caciocavallo cheese and prosciutto, sage and spices, sautéed and finished with white wine cream sauce and a hint of Marsala. I ask the waitperson to ask the chef to prepare the chicken without prosciutto.

Vitellina Alla Piemontese – Tender veal scaloppini over fresh spinach, topped with Fontina and prosciutto. I ask the waitperson to prepare the veal without the prosciutto.

Vitellina Alla Pizzaiola – Tender veal scaloppini sautéed with San Maranzo tomatoes, black olives and capers. Served over thin toast points and Pecorino Romano. I ask the waitperson to ask the chef to leave off the toast points.

Filetto Ai Ferri – Our beef tenderloin spends 7 days in a Chianti and fresh herb marinade, is grilled to your liking and finished with a porcini ragout.

Costolette Di Agnello – New Zeeland lamb chops roasted with a light Dijon & bread crumb coating. Served with a classic mint demi glaze. I ask the waitperson to ask the chef to leave off the bread crumbs.

Sides:

Broccolini – With Garlic and white wine.

Sautéed Spinach – With red onion and white wine.

Dolci:

Panna Cotta Trio – A trio of eggless custards: Madagascar vanilla bean, Bourbon and fresh orange, semi-sweet chocolate served with fresh berries.

Amaretti Al Forno – Almond cream and fresh berries fricassee topped with toasted Amaretti cookies.

Tiramisu – Strawberry covered tiramisu sprinkled with aged balsamic syrup.

Spumoni – Chocolate, pistachio and cherry ice cream served with fresh berries.

Goldie's Patio Grill
Tulsa, OK

Lite Side:

Chopped Sirloin Steak – Charbroiled to order. Served with cottage cheese, lettuce and tomato. I ask the waitperson to ask the chef to substitute extra lettuce and tomato for the cottage cheese.

Chicken Plate – Charbroiled chicken breast with cottage cheese, lettuce and tomato. I ask the waitperson to ask the chef to substitute extra lettuce and tomato for the cottage cheese.

Grilled Chicken Salad – Tender breast of chicken atop mixed greens, cheese & tomato.

House Salad – Tossed mixed greens with diced tomatoes, croutons & shredded cheddar jack cheese. I ask the waitperson to ask the chef to substitute extra diced tomatoes for the croutons.

Bowl of Chili

Hall of Flame Burgers:

We charbroil all of our burgers medium, medium well or well done. Served with one side item. You may substitute a dinner salad for an additional charge.

Goldie's Cheeseburger – Our fresh ground beef seasoned & cooked to order with cheese.

Goldie's Special – The original Goldie's burger cooked to order.

Hickory & Cheddar Jack Burger – With hickory sauce & cheddar Jack cheese.

Angel Fire Burger – Topped with melted cheddar Jack cheese & mild green chili pepper, served with picante.

Mushroom & Swiss Burger – Topped with sautéed mushrooms & Swiss cheese.

Chili & Cheese Burger – Open faced, covered with chili & American cheese. I ask the waitperson to ask the chef to substitute cheddar Jack cheese for the American cheese.

Patty Melt – Served on toasted rye and covered with Swiss cheese and grilled onions.

The "Cheesiest" Cheeseburger – Double the cheese for cheese lovers.

Side Items:

Slaw

Green Beans

Chili

Dinner Salad

Goldie's Platters:

All of our platters are served with Texas toast and your choice of two side items: slaw or green beans. I ask the waitperson to ask the chef to leave off the Texas toast.

The Ribeye – 10 oz. of tender steak that is seasoned and charbroiled to order.

Goldie's Dinner – Charburger steak stuffed with cheese & diced onion. Can add chili for an extra charge.

Angel Fire Dinner – Charburger steak stuffed with cheese & onions, topped with melted cheddar Jack cheese & a green chili pepper. Served with picante.

Mushroom Swiss Dinner – Charburger steak stuffed with cheese & diced onion then topped with sautéed mushrooms and Swiss cheese.

Hickory & Cheddar Jack Platter – Charburger steak stuffed with cheese & diced onions, with hickory sauce & melted cheddar Jack cheese.

Chicken Breast Platter – Tender, charbroiled, boneless chicken breast.

BBQ Chicken Breast Platter – Specially seasoned charbroiled boneless chicken breast topped with Goldie's hickory sauce.

Mushroom Swiss Chicken Breast Platter – Tender charbroiled boneless chicken breast topped with sautéed mushrooms and Swiss cheese.

Angel Fire Chicken Platter – Charbroiled chicken breast topped with a green chili pepper & melted cheddar Jack cheese.

Sandwiches:

All of our sandwiches are served on a toasted bun with one side item. Can substitute a side salad for an additional charge.

Charbroiled Chicken Sandwich – Tender charbroiled chicken breast.

BBQ Chicken Sandwich – Charbroiled chicken breast with Goldie's hickory sauce.

Angel Fire Chicken Sandwich – Charbroiled chicken breast with cheddar Jack cheese & a mild green chili pepper. Served with picante.

Mushroom & Swiss Chicken Sandwich – Charbroiled chicken breast topped with sautéed mushrooms and Swiss cheese.

Stuffed Charburger Sandwich – Hamburger steak filled with cheese and diced onions on Texas toast.

Ribeye Steak Sandwich – A 6 oz. cut, charbroiled with our special seasoning. Add Swiss cheese & sautéed mushrooms for an additional charge.

Houlihan's
Chain Restaurant

Apps + Shareable:

White Bean & Artichoke Hummus – With grilled pita, kalamata olives & basil oil.

Spicy Chicken and Avocado Eggrolls – Served with sour cream & house salsa.

Classic Spinach Dip – With cheesy lavosh crackers.

Houlihan's Famous 'Mushrooms – Panko crusted and garlic-herb cream cheese stuffed mushrooms with creamy horseradish sauce.

Chipotle Chicken Nachos – Chili roasted chicken, pepper jack, cheddar and chipotle cheese sauce, jalapenos, tomato, cilantro, guacamole, sour cream, house salsa. I ask the waitperson to ask the chef to substitute extra tomato for the jalapenos and guacamole.

Chicken Lettuce Wraps – Sweet and savory sesame glazed chicken, carrots, scallions and crispy wontons, peanut ginger sauce. I ask the waitperson to ask the chef to substitute extra carrots for the crispy wontons.

Sliders:

Veggie Mini Burger – Black bean and roasted vegetable patty topped with aged cheddar and ranch-style greens. I ask the waitperson to ask the chef to substitute extra greens for the black beans.

Pot Roast – With red wine mushroom gravy and crispy fried onions. I ask the waitperson to ask the chef to substitute grilled or sautéed onions for the crispy fried onions.

Creekstone Farms Black Angus Mini Burger – With aged cheddar & ranch-style greens.

Flatbreads:

Margherita Flatbread – Roma tomatoes, basil, fresh mozzarella, marinara.

Wild Mushroom & Arugula Flatbread – Crimini, shiitake & oyster mushrooms, roasted garlic white sauce, blend of cheeses & truffle vinaigrette.

BBQ Chicken Flatbread – Red onions, cilantro, pepper jack, Romano and cheddar cheese, sour cream drizzle.

Handhelds:

Add a bowl of homemade soup or side salad for an additional charge.

Brentwood Chicken Sandwich – Applewood smoked bacon, gouda cheese, Dijon mayo, baby greens, tomato & red onion on a buttered, toasted bun with choice of side. I ask the waitperson to ask the chef to substitute extra tomato for the bacon.

Southwest Grilled Chicken Wrap – Spicy pecans, red peppers, bacon, tortilla straws, pepper jack, garlic ranch, chips & house salsa. I ask the waitperson to ask the chef to substitute extra red peppers for the bacon and tortilla straws.

French Dip – Slow roasted and thin-sliced Angus roast beef, Swiss cheese on a toasted baguette with au jus and horseradish mayo, choice of side.

Taos Chipotle Turkey Wrap – Smoked turkey, guacamole, pepper Jack cheese, cilantro, lettuce, tomato & chipotle dressing. I ask the waitperson to ask the chef to substitute extra tomato for the guacamole.

Veggie Burger – Black bean and roasted vegetable patty topped with aged cheddar and ranch-style greens. I ask the waitperson to ask the chef to substitute extra greens for the black beans.

Creekstone Farms Black Angus Burger – (8oz.) A great burger starts with great beef. We take fresh Black Angus beef from Creekstone Farms, hand-form our burger patties in house and grill to your preferred temp. Served with crisp lettuce, tomato and red onion on a buttered, toasted bun with choice of side. Add for an additional charge sautéed mushrooms or cheese (aged cheddar, Swiss, gorgonzola, gouda or provolone). BBQ sauce available upon request.

Burger 72 – Topped with our famous –since 1972, garlic herb cream cheese-stuffed mushroom cap, horseradish sauce, parmesan and watercress.

Entrée Salads:

Add a bowl of homemade soup for an additional charge.

Spinach Salad – Toasted hazelnuts, kiwi, fresh berries & poppyseed dressing. For an additional charge can add goat cheese, thin-shaved chicken, or both.

Organic Power Greens Salad with Grilled Chicken – Toasted almonds, blueberries, blackberries, strawberries, goat cheese, poppyseed dressing, organic baby kale-spinach-chard blend.

Heartland Grilled Chicken Salad – Applewood smoked bacon, sharp aged cheddar, spicy pecans, red peppers, tomatoes, red onions, croutons, garlic ranch. I ask the waitperson to ask the chef to substitute extra red peppers and tomatoes for the smoked bacon and the croutons.

Chicken Asian Chop Chop – Sautéed sesame-glazed chicken, Napa salad, snow peas, roasted peanuts, red bell peppers, jicama, crispy wontons, peanut-ginger dressing. I ask the waitperson to ask the chef to substitute extra snow peas for the crispy wontons.

Buffalo Bleu Salad- Buffalo chicken tenders, Applewood smoked bacon, sharp cheddar, croutons, spicy pecans, red bell peppers, tomatoes, red onions, gorgonzola, garlic ranch. I ask the waitperson to ask the chef to substitute grilled chicken for the fried chicken tenders and to substitute extra red bell peppers and tomatoes for the bacon and croutons.

Chicken Caesar Salad – Grilled herb-marinated chicken breast, chopped romaine, Romano cheese, warm polenta croutons, and Caesar dressing. I ask the waitperson to ask the chef to substitute extra romaine for the croutons and to substitute bleu cheese dressing for the Caesar dressing.

Steak & Wedge Salad – (5oz.) sirloin, served with an iceberg wedge, smoked bacon, spicy pecans, roasted golden beets, grilled asparagus, gorgonzola, scallions, warm polenta croutons, and bleu cheese dressing. I ask the waitperson to ask the chef to substitute extra asparagus and scallions for the bacon and polenta croutons.

Premium Black Angus Steaks:

Our premium Black Angus aged steaks are hand-selected for dense marbling and hand-trimmed for superior cuts. All of our fresh beef is Midwestern raised, grain fed and aged a minimum of 28 days. All steaks are served with a bowl of our homemade soup or side salad and your choice of two sides.

Top Sirloin – 9 OZ. Top sirloin or 5 oz. Petite top sirloin.

Barrel-cut Filet Mignon – The juiciest, center-of-the-center cut filet for optimal flavor. The 6 oz. center-cut filet mignon. Or the 4 oz. petite center-cut filet mignon.

Classic Kansas City Strip – The 12 oz. grain fed KC strip.

Greens:

Tuscan White Bean Salad – With goat cheese, tomatoes, balsamic and Tuscan toast. I do not eat the toast.

Chop Salad – With bacon, corn, croutons, choice of bleu or cheddar and ranch or balsamic vinaigrette. I ask the waitperson to ask the chef to substitute extra bleu cheese for the bacon and croutons.

Spinach Salad – Toasted hazelnuts, kiwi, fresh berries, and poppyseed dressing.

Soup Kitchen:

Chicken Tortilla Soup – I ask the waitperson to ask the chef to leave off the tortilla strips.

Soup of the Day

Mains:

Add a bowl of homemade soup or side salad for an additional charge

Thai Grilled Chicken – Spicy-sweet grilled chicken served with pineapple brown rice, grilled asparagus and sesame-ginger soy. I ask the waitperson to ask the chef to substitute extra asparagus for the pineapple brown rice.

Stuffed Chicken Breast – Crisp, panko-breaded chicken breast stuffed with garlic-herb cream cheese, served with choice of vegetable and honest gold mashers. I ask the waitperson to ask the chef to leave the breading off my chicken and to substitute extra vegetables for the gold mashers.

Crispy Chicken Tenders – With French fries, choice of vegetable and honey mustard sub grilled chicken. I order the honey mustard grilled chicken and ask the waitperson to ask the chef to substitute an extra vegetable for the French fries.

Chicken Fettuccine Alfredo – Garlic and herb-marinated grilled chicken over fettuccine in a rich, buttery cream sauce with fontina, provolone and grated Romano.

Chicken Parmesan -Herb-crusted, sautéed chicken breast topped with marinara, fontina, provolone and Romano cheeses over fettuccine.

Down Home Angus Beef Pot Roast – Honest gold mashers, home-style vegetables, crispy fried onions and red wine mushroom gravy. I ask the waitperson to ask the chef to substitute grilled onions for the crispy fried onions and to substitute broccolini for the gold mashers.

Creekstone Farms Meatloaf – Black Angus beef meatloaf over honest gold mashers, crispy fried onions, red wine mushroom gravy and choice of vegetable. I order green beans. I ask the waitperson to ask the chef to substitute grilled onions for the crispy fried onions and to substitute broccolini for the gold mashers.

Desserts:

Grande Cappuccino Cake – A Houlihan's original from the 70s—#throwbackcappcake! Layers of rich chocolate cake with espresso icing and chocolate ganache, served with coffee ice cream, Kahlua fudge and caramel sauce.

White Chocolate Banana Cream Pie – Fresh bananas, pastry cream, caramel drizzle, and white chocolate shavings.

Bourbon Pecan Pie – Caramel and Cointreau Chantilly cream.

Italian Villa
Pasta & Pizza Restaurant
Anna, TX

Appetizers:

Stuffed Mushrooms

Mozzarella Caprese

Soup & Salads:

Tossed House Salad

Villa Salad- Lettuce, tomato, mushrooms, olives and mozzarella cheese.

Antipasto Salad – Lettuce, tomato, black olives, peppers, ham, salami & provolone cheese. I ask the waitperson to ask the chef to substitute extra tomato and lettuce for the ham.

Caesar – Can add chicken for an additional charge. I ask the waitperson to ask the chef to substitute Italian dressing for the Caesar dressing and to leave off the croutons.

Mediterranean Salad – Romaine tossed with roasted red peppers, artichokes, onions and feta cheese.

Minestrone Soup

Italian Tomato Soup

Neapolitan Pizza:

Toppings: Hamburger, mushrooms, onions, green pepper, black olives and extra cheese. Gourmet toppings: Artichoke, roasted red peppers, broccoli, pineapple, asparagus, chicken and ricotta can be added for an additional charge.

Cheese Pizza

Spinach Pizza

Pizza by the Slice

Hot Subs & Pizza Pockets:

Spinach Calzone

Philly Steak

Homemade Pastas:

All pastas are served with homemade garlic rolls.

Pasta Sampler – Manicotti, cannelloni & lasagna.

Baked Eggplant Rollatini

Manicotti

Cannelloni

Baked Tortellini – Choice of beef or cheese.

Baked Ziti

Lasagna

Stuffed Shells

Spaghetti – Choice of tomato sauce, meat sauce, meatballs, or mushrooms.

Entrees:

All entrees are served with tossed salad and house-made garlic rolls.

Rigatoni or Capellini Pomodoro – Sautéed garlic with diced tomatoes, onions, fresh basil, and a touch of marinara, tossed with angel hair or rigatoni pasta.

Chicken Aristocrat – Boneless breast of chicken sautéed in a white cream sauce with a touch of marinara, topped with eggplant and mozzarella cheese.

Chicken Diane – Boneless breast of chicken sautéed with artichokes, mushrooms and onions in a white wine cream sauce with a touch of marinara. Served with spaghetti.

Chicken Alfredo – Boneless breast of chicken with fettuccini in Alfredo sauce.

Chicken Murphy – Boneless breast of chicken sautéed with fresh red peppers, mushrooms, onions and jalapenos in a white wine cream sauce with a touch of marinara. Served with spaghetti. I ask the waitperson to ask the chef to prepare my chicken without jalapenos.

Chicken Cacciatore – Boneless breast of chicken with fresh red and green peppers, mushrooms, onions and fresh garlic in a white wine marinara sauce. Served with spaghetti.

Chicken Scarparelli – Chicken breast sautéed with mushrooms, red peppers, scallions and garlic in a white cream sauce, then topped with mozzarella cheese, baked and served over a bed of spaghetti.

Chicken Florentine – Boneless breast of chicken sliced with spinach and sautéed mushrooms in a white cream sauce. Served with fettuccini.

Chicken Giusseppe – Boneless breast of chicken sautéed with mushrooms, scallions and fresh garlic in a Marsala wine sauce with a touch of marinara. Served with spaghetti.

Chicken Marsala – Boneless breast of chicken with sautéed mushrooms, in a Marsala wine sauce. Served with spaghetti.

Chicken Piccata – Boneless breast of chicken with a white wine and lemon butter sauce with capers. Served with spaghetti.

Chicken Adamo – Chicken breast sautéed with sun-dried tomato and artichokes in a lemon-basil sauce, served with angel hair pasta.

Chicken Maximo – Chicken breast sautéed with sun-dried tomatoes, asparagus, fresh tomato, mushrooms and melted mozzarella in a light red wine sauce, served with a side of spaghetti.

Veal Entrees

Veal Piccata

Veal Murphy

Veal Giusseppe

Veal Marsala

House Specials:

Tortellini alla Vodka – Cheese filled tortellini pasta tossed with broccoli and roasted red pepper in a Vodka cream sauce.

Rigatoni alla Pesto – Rigatoni pasta tossed with artichoke, roasted red peppers and garlic in a basil pesto sauce.

Additional Items:

Meatballs

Breast of Chicken

Side of Tomato Sauce

John E's
Louisville, KY

Lunch:

Salads:

Specialty Tossed Salad

Elizabeth's Chef Salad – I ask the waitperson to ask the chef to substitute turkey for the ham.

Baby Spinach Salad – I ask the waitperson to ask the chef to leave off the bacon.

Chicken Salad

Peachy Romaine Salad

Soup and Salad

Sandwiches:

John E's Steak Burger with Cheese

Sliced Turkey & Bacon – on Tomato basil focaccia. I ask the waitperson to ask the chef to substitute extra lettuce and tomato for the bacon.

Hot Roast Beef

Chicken Salad on a Roll

Pepper Steak Sandwich

Entrees:

8 oz. Ribeye Steak

Petite Filet Mignon

Chopped Sirloin

Celestial Chicken

Charbroiled Chicken

Dinner:

Salads:

Special Tossed Salad

Peachy Romaine Salad

Entrees:

2 lb. T-bone

2 lb. T-bone for 2

New York Strip

Prime Filet Mignon

Ribeye Pepper Steak

Cowboy Ribeye

Petite Filet Steak

Charbroiled Chicken

Celestial Chicken

Steak Burger

Compliments:

Today's Vegetable

Coleslaw

Dinner Salad

Buttered Mushroom Caps

Desserts:

John E's Black Bottom Pie

Derby Pie

Chocolate Chocolate Cake

Carrot Cake

Luigi's Italian Restaurant
Atoka, OK

Salads:

Choice of Dressings: House Italian, Ranch, Oil & Vinegar, Balsamic Vinegar. Chicken can be added for an additional charge.

Tossed Salad – Fresh iceberg lettuce, tomatoes, and cheese.

Luigi Salad – Fresh lettuce topped with black olives, mushrooms, and mozzarella cheese.

Caesar Salad – Fresh romaine lettuce tossed with homemade Caesar dressing, croutons, and parmesan cheese. I ask the waitperson to ask the chef to leave off the croutons and to substitute House Italian for the Caesar dressing.

Roma Salad – Fresh lettuce, tomato, garlic, cheese, artichoke hearts, bell peppers, mushrooms, capers, black olives, and tossed in lemon sauce.

Sandwiches:

I eat the bread on a reward day.

Veggie Stromboli – Peppers, onion, mushrooms, black olives, served with marinara sauce wrapped in pizza crust.

Meatball Parmigiana Sub – Baked French bread topped with meatballs, marinara sauce and mozzarella cheese.

Philly Cheese Steak – Baked French bread topped with sautéed onions, green peppers, mushrooms, mozzarella cheese, and steak pieces.

Baked Pasta:

I eat pasta dishes on a reward night.

Lasagna – Pasta layered with beef, mozzarella cheese topped

with marinara sauce and mozzarella cheese.

Manicotti – Pasta stuffed and rolled with ricotta cheese, topped with marinara sauce and mozzarella cheese.

Pasta Sampler – Lasagna, manicotti, and eggplant topped with marinara sauce and mozzarella cheese.

Pastas:

I eat pasta on a reward night.

Spaghetti with Meatballs

Spaghetti with Meat Sauce

Spaghetti with Mushrooms

Tortellini Modo Mio with Chicken – Cheese tortellini pasta and chicken sautéed with basil, tomatoes, broccoli, and garlic in a white wine sauce with marinara.

House Specials:

On non-reward days I ask the waitperson to ask the chef to substitute broccoli or green beans for the pasta.

Luigi Special – Grilled chicken breast and sausage sautéed with roasted red bell peppers, ham and black olives in a white wine, cream sauce with a touch of marinara sauce served over fettuccini pasta. I ask the waitperson to ask the chef to substitute extra chicken for sausage and ham.

Chicken Broccoli – Fettuccini pasta served with chicken and broccoli in a cream sauce.

Chicken Damabianka – Grilled chicken breast sautéed with fresh mushrooms in a white cream sauce and served over spaghetti pasta.

Chicken Aristocrat – Grilled chicken breast topped with eggplant and provolone cheese, sautéed in sherry wine, cream sauce with a touch of marinara sauce.

Chicken Tetrazzini – Grilled chicken breast sautéed red bell peppers with white wine, cream sauce with a touch of marinara sauce over spaghetti pasta.

Chicken Genovese – Grilled chicken topped with asparagus, provolone cheese, sautéed in white wine, cream sauce and a touch of marinara sauce, served over spaghetti pasta.

Chicken Carchovi – Grilled chicken breast sautéed with artichoke hearts and mushrooms in a creamy white sauce, served over spaghetti pasta.

Pasta Primavera with Chicken – Fettuccini pasta sautéed with fresh mixed vegetables, grilled chicken in a cream sauce with a touch of marinara sauce.

Chicken Capellini – Grilled chicken sautéed in olive oil, garlic, basil, artichoke hearts and fresh vegetables in white wine sauce, over spaghetti pasta with a touch of marinara sauce.

Chicken Marsala – Grilled chicken breast sautéed with mushrooms, Marsala wine, with a touch of red sauce over spaghetti pasta.

Chicken Florentine – Grilled chicken breast sautéed with spinach, mushrooms, garlic, white wine, cream sauce over fettuccini pasta.

Chicken Pomodoro – Grilled chicken sautéed with fresh tomatoes, basil, olive oil, garlic, sherry wine, marinara sauce served over penne pasta.

Chicken Siciliano – Grilled chicken breasts sautéed with mushrooms, artichoke hearts, in a white wine lemon sauce, served over spaghetti pasta.

Chicken Piccata – Grilled chicken breast sautéed with capers in a white wine, lemon sauce, served over spaghetti pasta.

<u>Chicken Cacciatore</u> – Grilled chicken sautéed with fresh mushrooms, onions, green peppers in a marinara sauce served with spaghetti pasta.

<u>Desserts:</u>

<u>Triple Chocolate Cheesecake</u>

<u>Tiramisu</u>

The Mediterranean Grill
Chesterfield, MO

Appetizers:

Falafel Balls – Five freshly cooked falafel balls served with tehina sauce.

Dips n' Spreads Sampler Plate – Carrot salad, eggplant spread, matbocha (Moroccan salsa, and Middle Eastern chopped vegetable salad) served with pita bread. Sampler Plate does not include hummus.

Soup de Jour

Salads:

Greek Salad – Lettuce, tomatoes, cucumber, onion, Kalamata olives and feta cheese served with our special Greek dressing. I ask the waitperson to ask the chef to substitute extra tomatoes for the cucumbers.

House Gorgonzola Salad – Spring mix lettuce, cherry tomatoes, cucumber, carrots, raisins, onions, pine nuts and crumbled gorgonzola in a special house vinaigrette dressing. I ask the waitperson to ask the chef to substitute extra lettuce for the cucumbers.

Mediterranean Salad – Chopped tomatoes, cucumbers, onions, cilantro, chick peas and hardboiled egg on a bed of spinach leaves. I ask the waitperson to ask the chef to substitute extra tomatoes for the cucumbers.

Signature Platters:

Falafel – Vegetable patties made from chickpeas, parsley, onion, cilantro, and spices served with Mediterranean salad, humus, and pita.

Chicken Souvlaki – Grilled boneless chicken breast topped with tzatziki sauce and feta cheese. Add a Greek salad for an additional charge.

Gyro – Greek spiced meat topped with Tzatzki sauce and feta cheese. Add a Greek salad for an additional charge.

House Specialties:

Each of the items below is served on a platter that includes couscous or sliced baked potatoes. Add three sampler size dips n' spreads for an additional charge.

Stuffed Eggplant – Spiced ground beef mixed with cilantro and parsley, wedged between two eggplant slices and baked to perfection.

Lamb with Apricots and Prunes – Lamb baked with onions, prunes and raisins.

Moroccan Meatballs with Peas – Ground beef meatballs cooked with peas and seasoned with Moroccan spices.

Schnitzel Platter – Pan fried chicken breast.

Vegetarian Stuffed Peppers – Bell peppers stuffed with rice, carrots, apricots, raisins and spices and served with a side of falafel balls.

From the Grill:

Each of the items below is served on a platter that includes couscous or sliced baked potatoes, as well as sampler sized dips n' spreads for an additional charge.

Elie's Mix – Stir-fried cubes of boneless chicken breast, sirloin, potato, onion, and spices.

Italian Style Chicken Kabob – Two skewers of grilled chicken cubes marinated in wine, garlic, and thyme.

Spanish Style Shish Kabob – Two skewers of sirloin cubes marinated in wine and onions.

Lamb Kabob – Two skewers of spiced lamb cubes.

Middle Eastern Style Ground Lamb & Beef Kofte Kabob – Lamb and beef mixed with onions, garlic, and parsley.

Desserts:

Baklava

Cream Bavaria

Mimi's Café
New Menu
Chain Restaurant

Appetizers:

French Onion Soup – I ask the waitperson to ask the chef to prepare it without any bread or croutons.

Tomato Basil

Chef's Choice

Craft Sandwiches:

With your choice of fresh-cut fruit or a Mimi's House Salad unless otherwise noted. Can substitute a cup of soup for an additional charge.

Roasted Turkey & Brie Melt – Hand-carved, house-roasted turkey with crisp green apple on a fresh-baked, all-butter croissant. Served with a side of apricot chutney.

French Dip – Sliced roast beef on a fresh baguette with horseradish cream and a side of au jus. Add bell peppers, caramelized onions, mushrooms and mozzarella for an additional charge.

Grilled Chicken Sandwich – On a fresh-baked multigrain croissant with mixed greens, fresh tomatoes and basil-pesto mayonnaise.

Can add Jack, Swiss, cheddar, blue, or mozzarella cheese to sandwiches for an additional charge.

Café Sandwiches.

With your choice of fresh-cut fruit or a Mimi's House Salad unless otherwise noted. Can substitute a cup of soup for an additional charge.

Chicken Salad Croissant – Grilled tarragon chicken salad with red grapes and walnuts on a fresh-baked, multigrain croissant. I do not eat the grapes.

Roasted Turkey Club – Triple decker of hand-carved, house-roasted turkey, hickory-smoked bacon, lettuce, tomatoes and mayonnaise on toasted sourdough. I ask the waitperson to ask the chef to leave off the center slice of bread and to substitute extra tomatoes for the bacon.

Burgers:

With your choice of fresh-cut fruit or a Mimi's House Salad unless otherwise noted. Can substitute a cup of soup for an additional charge.

Brioche Cheeseburger – On a toasted brioche bun with lettuce, tomatoes, red onions, pickles, Thousand Island Dressing and your choice of cheese. I ask the waitperson to ask the chef to substitute Dijon mustard for the Thousand Island Dressing.

Salads:

With a petite French Baguette or fresh-baked muffin. I do not eat the bread.

Mediterranean Salad with Roasted Chicken – Crispy prosciutto, tomatoes, cucumbers, Kalamata olives, roasted red peppers, red onions, artichoke hearts, pepperoncini and feta cheese with mixed greens. Served with red wine shallot vinaigrette. I ask the waitperson to ask the chef to substitute extra tomatoes and mixed greens for the cucumbers and prosciutto.

Grilled Chicken Caesar – With chopped hearts of romaine, grated parmesan and black pepper croutons. Served with Caesar Dressing. I ask the waitperson to ask the chef to leave off the croutons and to substitute bleu cheese dressing for the Caesar dressing.

Tomato & Mozzarella – Sliced summer tomatoes, buffalo mozzarella, and cherry tomatoes. Sprinkled with chopped fresh basil and served with balsamic vinaigrette.

Bacon & Bleu Cheese – Hickory-smoked bacon, walnuts, crumbled bleu cheese, tomatoes, and dried cranberries tossed with mixed greens. Topped with fresh strawberries. Grilled chicken can be added for an additional charge. I ask the waitperson to ask the chef to substitute extra strawberries for the bacon.

Chicken Chop Salad – Slow-roasted chicken breast, red & green bell peppers, mandarin orange slices, basil, cilantro, chopped cabbage and romaine lettuce. Served with sesame dressing, fried wontons and sesame seeds. I ask the waitperson to ask the chef to leave off the fried wontons.

Entrees:

Add Mimi's House Salad or a cup of soup for an additional charge. A bit of France.

Roasted Chicken Crepes – House-made crepes with slow-roasted chicken, sautéed spinach & mushrooms, and sliced cherry tomatoes topped with Dijon Chardonnay sauce. With a Mimi's House Salad tossed in red wine shallot vinaigrette.

Tenderloin Medallions – Two beef medallions with au gratin potatoes and your choice of a rich red wine or creamy béarnaise sauce and fresh vegetables. I ask the waitperson to ask the chef to substitute extra fresh vegetables for the potatoes.

Chef's Choice Quiche – With a freshly baked muffin and Mimi's House Salad.

Coq au Vin – Chicken braised in red wine, mushrooms and pearl onions. Served over mashed potatoes and peas. I ask the waitperson to ask the chef to substitute steamed broccoli for the potatoes.

Grilled Bistro Steak – Au gratin potatoes and your choice of a rich creamy béarnaise or red wine sauce and fresh vegetables. I ask the waitperson to ask the chef to substitute extra vegetables for the potatoes.

American Comfort:

Slow-Roasted Turkey – Hand-carved, house-roasted turkey with mashed potatoes, gravy, cornbread dressing, fresh vegetables and orange-apple cranberry relish. I ask the waitperson to ask the chef to substitute extra fresh vegetables for the potatoes and cornbread dressing.

Meatloaf & Mash – With creamy mashed potatoes, gravy and fresh vegetables. I asked the waitperson to ask the chef to substitute extra fresh vegetables for the mashed potatoes and gravy.

Beef Pot Roast – Slowly braised in a red wine shallot sauce. Served with creamy mashed potatoes and fresh vegetables. I ask the waitperson to ask the chef to substitute extra fresh vegetables for the mashed potatoes.

Desserts:

Brioche Bread Pudding – with Bourbon-butter sauce.

Triple Chocolate Brownie – Served warm with vanilla bean ice cream and chocolate and caramel sauce.

The Old Spaghetti Factory
Chain Restaurant

Enjoy Our Complete Meal!

All of our entrees come with fresh baked bread, soup or crisp green salad with a choice of dressing, coffee, hot tea, iced tea, or milk and our signature spumoni ice cream for dessert.

Entrée Salads:

BLT Salad – Chopped hearts of romaine tossed with blue cheese dressing, croutons and crisp bacon, served with diced Roma tomatoes, avocados and garnished with blue cheese crumbles. I ask the waitperson to ask the chef to substitute extra romaine and tomatoes for the bacon, croutons, and avocados.

Chicken Caesar Salad – Lightly breaded, all-natural chicken breast strips atop crisp romaine lettuce tossed with classic Caesar dressing, shredded Romano cheese, garlic herb croutons, and Roma tomatoes. Also available without chicken.

I ask the waitperson to ask the chef to prepare my chicken without breading. I also request that extra romaine lettuce be substituted for the croutons and blue cheese dressing be substituted for the Caesar dressing.

Signature Selections:

Angel Hair Pomodoro – Diced tomatoes simmered with fresh onions, garlic and basil. Served over a bed of angel hair pasta, garnished with fresh basil and topped with shredded Romano cheese.

Chicken Penne – Slices of all-natural chicken breast with Marinara and Alfredo sauces over penne noodles topped with shredded Romano cheese.

Baked Chicken – (Available for Dinner only) Baked breast of all-natural chicken marinated in garlic and lemon juice, seasoned with oregano, served with spaghetti, Mizithra Cheese & Browned Butter and Marinara sauce. I ask the waitperson to ask the chef to substitute Angel Hair Pomodoro for the Mizithra Cheese & Browned Butter and Marinara sauce.

Pasta Classics:

Our Sauces: All of our sauces are made daily in our own kitchen with the finest ingredients available. Pasta-bilities: All dishes are served with the finest 100% durum semolina spaghetti or whole wheat pasta. Gluten free available.

Rich Meat Sauce – Ground beef sautéed with onions and celery then simmered with tomatoes and Italian spices.

Mushroom Sauce – Our Marinara sauce topped with sautéed mushrooms.

Marinara Sauce – Fresh onions and garlic simmered with diced tomatoes, red wine and Italian seasonings.

Sicilian Meatballs – Two large roasted beef meatballs delicately seasoned then topped with Marinara sauce.

Factory Favorites:

Chicken Parmigiana – A seasoned breast of all-natural chicken topped with melted cheese and Marinara served with spaghetti Marinara. I ask the waitperson to ask the chef to leave the breading off the chicken and to substitute broccoli for the spaghetti.

Breast of Chicken Fettuccini – Fettuccini topped with breast of all-natural chicken strips, fresh broccoli and mushrooms and covered with Alfredo sauce.

Chicken Marsala – A seasoned breast of all-natural chicken with a fresh mushroom and Marsala wine sauce, served alongside spaghetti with Mizithra Cheese & browned butter. I ask the waitperson to ask the chef to substitute broccoli for the Mizithra Cheese & brown butter spaghetti.

Spinach & Cheese Ravioli – Tender pillows of pasta stuffed with spinach and two kinds of cheese, and topped with our savory Marinara sauce.

Sides:

Fresh Broccoli – Broccoli lightly flavored with Mizithra cheese and browned butter. I ask the waitperson to ask the chef to prepare the broccoli either steamed or without the cheese and browned butter. For an additional cost broccoli can be substituted for pasta.

Side of Meatballs

Desserts:

Mud Pie – A rich chocolate cookie crust filled with mocha almond fudge ice cream, topped with almonds and chocolate syrup.

Lunch For Less:

Lunch-sized Pasta entries served with hot fresh baked bread and soup or a crisp green salad with choice of dressing.

Pasta Classic Entrees:

See dinner menu above for pasta choices.

Lunch-Sized Salads:

See dinner menu above for salad choices.

Soup & Salad – (Dine-in Only) Crisp green salad served with soup of the day and hot baked bread.

Sandwiches:

Sandwiches are served with potato chips. Add soup or salad for an additional charge. I do not eat the potato chips.

Chicken & Smoked Mozzarella Panini – Grilled, all-natural chicken breast, smoked mozzarella, sun-dried tomatoes and bacon on a rustic Italian bread spread with pesto aioli, then grilled Panini style. I ask the waitperson to ask the chef to leave off the bacon.

Reuben Panini – Our version of the classic Reuben sandwich grilled Panini style on fresh dark rye bread filled with delicious sauerkraut, tender corned beef, Swiss cheese and our own 1000 Island dressing. I ask the waitperson to ask the chef to substitute mustard for the 1000 Island dressing.

Ham & Cheddar Panini – Slices of honey ham and cheddar cheese with Dijon aioli spread on rustic Italian bread, grilled Panini style. I ask the waitperson to ask the chef to substitute the all-natural chicken breast for the ham.

Half Sandwich with Soup of Salad – Choose your favorite sandwich served with potato chips and either soup or salad.

Outback Steakhouse
International Chain Restaurant

Ausssie-Tizers® To Share:

Alice Springs Chicken Quesadillas ® Stuffed with fresh grilled chicken breast, sautéed mushrooms, bacon, melted cheeses and honey mustard sauce. I ask the waitperson to ask the chef to prepare my quesadillas without bacon.

Chicken Artichoke Flatbread – Crispy flatbread topped with wood-fire grilled chicken, chopped spinach, artichokes and Parmesan cheese.

Spinach Artichoke Dip – A creamy blend of spinach, artichokes, Monterey Jack and Parmesan baked until bubbly. Served with White corn tortilla chips. I do not eat the tortilla chips.

Soups & Salads:

Walkabout Soup ® Of The Day – Today's fresh made soup.

French Onion Soup – Made with our world-famous onions and topped with melted Provolone cheese. I ask the waitperson to ask the chef to prepare the soup without bread.

Aussie Chicken Cobb Salad – Wood-fired grilled or crispy chicken, fresh mixed greens, chopped hard-boiled eggs, tomatoes, bacon, Monterey Jack and Cheddar cheese and freshly made croutons. Tossed in your choice of dressing. I order the wood-fired grilled chicken. I ask the waitperson to ask the chef to substitute extra mixed greens for the bacon and croutons.

Sesame Salad – Grilled chicken, mixed greens, red peppers, chopped cilantro, sliced almonds and sesame seeds tossed in sesame vinaigrette.

Steakhouse Salad – Seared sirloin, mixed greens, Aussie

Crunch, tomatoes, red onions, cinnamon pecans and Danish Blue Cheese vinaigrette. I ask the waitperson to ask the waiter to substitute extra mixed greens for the Aussie Crunch.

Chicken Caesar Salad – Wood-fire grilled chicken, crisp Romaine and freshly made croutons. Tossed in our Caesar dressing. I ask the waitperson to ask the chef to substitute extra Romaine for the croutons and to substitute Blue Cheese dressing for the Caesar dressing.

Steak Plates:

Served with Aussie Fries. Add a cup of Walkabout Soup, one of our Signature Side Salads, or one of our Premium Side Salads for an additional charge. I ask the waitperson to substitute a vegetable for the fries.

Sirloin with Wild Mushroom Sauce – Our 6 oz. signature sirloin topped with our rich Marsala and wild mushroom sauce.

Sirloin Diablo – Our 6 oz. signature sirloin topped with a zesty chili pepper cream sauce.

Burgers & Sandwiches:

Served with Aussie Fries. Add a cup of Walkabout Soup, one of our Signature Side Salads, or one of our Premium Side Salads for an additional charge. I ask the waitperson to substitute a vegetable for the fries.

The Outback Burger – Topped with lettuce, tomato, onion, pickle and mustard.

Classic Cheese Burger – Topped with your choice of cheese: Swiss, Provolone or Cheddar and lettuce, tomato, onion, pickle and mustard.

Double Burger – Two wood-fire grilled patties topped with American cheese, lettuce, tomato, red onion, and mayo on a grilled broche bun. I ask the waitperson to ask the chef to substitute cheddar or Swiss cheese for the American cheese.

Wood-Grilled California Chicken Sandwich – Topped with bacon, lettuce, tomato, lemon pepper aioli and avocado. I ask the waitperson to ask the chef to substitute extra tomatoes for the bacon and avocado.

Prime Rib Dip Sandwich – Thin-sliced seared prime rib with grilled onions and Swiss cheese.

Create Your Own Signature Steak:

Customize your steak experience by the following steps below. Signature steaks are cooked to order and served with your choice of a cup of Walkabout Soup or one of our Signature Side Salads and one freshly made side.

1. Choose your cut and size:

Outback Special® – Our signature sirloin is one of the leanest cuts, hearty and full of flavor. 6 oz., 8 oz., or 11 oz.

Victoria's Filet® – The most tender and juicy thick cut. 6 oz. or 8 oz.

Kansas City Strip – Full of rich flavor. 12 oz.

Ribeye – The steak lover's steak is well-marbled, juicy and savory. 10 oz. or 12 oz.

T-Bone – This T-bone is like two steaks in one – a flavorful strip and filet tenderloin together, seared for a juicy taste. 20.oz.

2. Choose Your Cooking Style:

Classic Seasoned & Seared or Wood-Fire Grilled

3. Choose Your Temperature:

4. Choose Your Soup or Salad & One Freshly Made Side:

Walkabout Soup® – Cup

Signature Side Salads

House Salad – I ask the waitperson to ask the chef to substitute extra lettuce for the cucumbers and croutons.

Caesar Salad – I ask the waitperson to ask the chef to substitute extra lettuce for the croutons and to substitute blue cheese dressing for the Caesar dressing.

Premium Side Salads for an additional charge

Classic Blue Cheese Wedge Salad

Blue Cheese Pecan Chopped Salad

Sides:

Fresh Steamed Broccoli

Fresh Steamed Green Beans

Fresh Seasonal Mixed Vegetables

Grilled Asparagus for an additional charge

5. Choose Your Add Ons:

Blue Cheese Crumb Crust

Horseradish Crumb Crust

Sautéed Mushrooms

Outback Favorites:

Add a coup of Walkabout Soup, one of our Signature Side Salads, or one of our Premium Salads for an additional charge.

Filet With Wild Mushroom Sauce – Wood-fire grilled petite filet topped with Marsala and wild mushroom sauce. Garlic mashed potatoes and fresh seasonal mixed veggies. I ask the waitperson to ask the chef to substitute extra mixed veggies for the potatoes.

New Zealand Lamb – Finished with a rich Cabernet wine sauce. Garlic mashed potatoes and fresh seasonal mixed veggies. I ask the waitperson to ask the chef to substitute extra mixed veggies for the potatoes.

Alice Springs Chicken® – Wood-fire chicken breast topped with sautéed mushrooms, crisp bacon, melted Monterey Jack and Cheddar and honey mustard sauce. Aussie Fries. I ask the waitperson to ask the chef to leave off the bacon and to substitute mixed veggies for the fries.

Specialty Cuts & Combos:

Add a coup of Walkabout Soup, one of our Signature Side Salads, or one of our Premium Salads for an additional charge.

Teriyaki Filet Medallions – Wood-fire grilled teriyaki marinated filet, onions, red and green peppers over seasoned rice. Choose two sides. I ask the waitperson to ask the chef to substitute extra onions and peppers for the rice.

Herb Roasted Prime Rib – (based on availability) Seasoned and slow-roasted prime rib. Hand-carved to order with traditional au jus. Choice of two sides. 8 oz., 12 oz., or 16 oz.

Freshly Made Sides:

See number 4 above.

Irresistible Desserts:

Sweet Adventure Sampler Trio® – Sample three fabulous desserts: Chocolate Thunder from Down Under® with pecan brownie, Carrot Cake with coconut and pecans and Classic Cheesecake. Or choose one individual portion.

Pan D' Olive
St. Louis, MO

Mezes:

Carpaccio – With shaved Parmigiano, arugula, and artichoke hearts.

Pan-Fried Eggplant – With tomato sauce.

Grilled Lamb Kofte – With yogurt, cucumber, tomato, and onion. I ask the waitperson to ask the chef to leave off the cucumber.

Marinated Olives – Orange zest, garlic, and herbs.

The Green Side:

Wedge Salad – with bacon, tomato, and blue cheese crumbles. I ask the waitperson to ask the chef to leave off the bacon.

Shepherd Salad – Cucumber, olive, tomato, onion, and feta. I ask the waitperson to ask the chef to substitute extra tomato for the cucumber.

Spinach Salad – With candied walnuts, cranberries, gorgonzola, and pomegranate vinaigrette. Chicken can be added for an additional charge.

Flatbreads:

Pan D' Olive – With chicken, mushroom, olive, gorgonzola, and caramelized onion.

Vendura – With asparagus, tomato, roasted peppers, feta, and balsamic onion.

Pasta:

Chicken Tortellini – With Mushrooms, peas, and tomatoes in sherry cream.

Capellini – With mushrooms, capers, Kalamata olives, and spicy tomato.

Entrees:

Sirloin Steak – With gorgonzola cream, grilled tomatoes, and mashed potatoes. I ask the waitperson to ask the chef to substitute asparagus for the potatoes.

Filet Mignon – Breaded, mozzarella, brandy mushrooms, and mashed potatoes. I ask the waitperson to ask the chef to leave off the breading and to substitute cabbage stew for the potatoes.

Chicken Madeira – With mushrooms, bell peppers, tomatoes, Madeira wine, and asparagus.

Rosemary Chicken – With garlic, white wine, lemon, and rice pilaf. I ask the waitperson to ask the chef to substitute spinach for the rice.

Turkish Specialties:

Kofte Iskender Kebab – Lamb Kofte, pita, marinara, yogurt. I ask the waitperson to ask the chef to substitute cabbage stew for the pita with yogurt.

Lamb Shank – Vegetable lamb jus, and rice pilaf. I ask the waitperson to ask the chef to substitute asparagus for the rice pilaf.

Imam Bayilid – Braised eggplant with ground beef stuffing.

Side Dishes:

Asparagus

Spinach

Cabbage Stew

Dessert:

Hazelnut Tiramisu

Baklava

Turtle Cheesecake

The Pasta House Co.
St. Louis, MO; Paducah, KY; Belleville, IL

Appetizers:

Nonna Tucci's Meatballs

Sicilian Stuffed Artichoke

Artichoke and Spinach Dip with Crostini

Portobello Fritto – Fresh Portobello mushrooms.

Salads & Soups:

The Pasta House Co. Special Salad – I ask the waitperson to ask the chef to leave off the croutons.

Soup of the Day – Fresh daily, refills available.

Minestrone Soup – Fresh daily, refills available. Classis Italian soup with hearty beef broth and fresh vegetables.

The "Best" Grilled Chicken Caesar – Romaine lettuce, grilled chicken and Caesar dressing. I ask the waitperson to ask the chef to leave off the croutons and to substitute Italian dressing for the Caesar dressing.

Sandwiches:

Served with French fries or pasta. Can add the Pasta House Co. Special Salad for an additional charge. I ask the waitperson to ask the chef to substitute the salad for the French fries on all sandwiches.

Roast Beef

Chicken Parmigiano – I ask the waitperson to ask the chef to substitute grilled chicken for the breaded chicken.

Chicken Portobello – Grilled chicken breast, sautéed mushrooms, fresh mozzarella and crispy onion strings. I ask the waitperson to ask the chef to substitute grilled or sautéed onions for the crispy onion strings.

Nonna Tucci's Meatball Sub – Topped with tomato sauce and onion on hot cheesy garlic bread.

Philly Cheesesteak Sub – Roast beef, green pepper and onion on hot cheesy garlic bread.

Lunch Menu:

All regular menu items also available at lunch. Lunch specials are not valid with any other offer or coupon. No substitutions please.

The Pasta House Co. Special Salad – Small or large.

Soup and The Pasta House Co. Special Salad

Mt. Vesuvius Hot Chicken Filets (1/2 lb.) and The Pasta House Co. Special Salad

House Specials:

Served with a side of pasta and your choice of soup or The Pasta House Co. Special Salad.

Nonna Tucci's Meatballs Parmigiano

Chicken Parmigiano (low calorie) – I ask the waitperson to ask the chef to prepare the chicken without breading.

Chicken Marsala (low calorie)

Mangia Bene (eat well):

Low fat, low calorie or low carb but still 110% Pasta House Co. fantastic. The following are served with The Pasta House Co. Special Salad. (Low fat Pasta House Co. dressing is available.)

Low calorie:

Grilled Chicken Breast – 6 oz. with steamed broccoli.

Chicken Rustico – Grilled chicken breast served in a tomato Marsala sauce with mushrooms, artichokes, capers and sundried tomatoes and served with steamed broccoli.

Pastas:

Tomato Sauce:

Spaghetti Bolognese – In our famous meat sauce.

Mostaccioli – In our famous meat sauce.

Spaghetti with Nonna Tucci's Meatballs

Penne Primavera – Quill shaped pasta with fresh zucchini, mushrooms and broccoli in a sundried tomato herb sauce.

Pastas with Chicken:

Chicken Ignatio (mangia bene) – Rigatoni in a tomato cream sauce with grilled chicken, roasted red peppers, mushrooms, peas and prosciutto. I ask the waitperson to ask the chef to prepare this dish without the prosciutto.

Pollo e Portobello (back by popular demand) – Linguine prepared with grilled chicken, sautéed mushrooms, prosciutto, shallots, white wine sauce and fresh sage. I ask the waitperson to ask the chef to prepare this dish without the prosciutto.

Penne Romano with Chicken Spiedini – Charcoal grilled breaded chicken spiedini served over penne noodles in tomato sauce with sundried tomato pesto. I ask the waitperson to ask the chef to prepare my chicken without the breading.

Chicken Fettuccine – Egg noodles prepared in a cream sauce with grilled chicken, peas, mushrooms and Parmigiano cheese.

Entrees:

All are served with The Pasta House Co. Special Salad and your choice of two: Pasta with Bolognese or Alfredo sauce, steamed broccoli or Italian potatoes. I order the steamed broccoli and Italian potatoes or a double order of steamed broccoli.

Chicken Flamingo – Grilled breast of chicken lightly breaded, served in a sauce of white wine, garlic, red peppers, broccoli, fresh mushrooms, prosciutto, mozzarella and provolone cheese. I ask the waitperson to ask the chef to prepare my Chicken Flamingo without the breading and without the prosciutto.

Chicken Marsala – Boneless breast of chicken lightly breaded, Marsala wine sauce, oregano, fresh green peppers and fresh mushrooms. I ask the waitperson to ask the chef to prepare my Chicken Marsala without the breading.

Chicken Rustico (mangia bene) – Grilled chicken breast served in a tomato Marsala sauce with mushrooms, artichokes, capers, and sun dried tomatoes and served with steamed broccoli.

Served with The Pasta House Co Special Salad:

Grilled Chicken Breasts (mangia bene) – 8 oz. charcoal grilled and served with steamed broccoli.

Pizza:

Cheese – 12" or 16 ".

Hamburger – 12" or 16".

Mushroom – 12" or 16".

Artichoke, Tomato and Basil – 12" or 16".

Green Pepper & Onion – 12" or 16".

Super Veggie – Sundried tomato, mushroom, artichoke, roasted zucchini, and red pepper.

Artichoke Dip Pizza – Topped with our signature artichoke dip and mixed cheese blend and more artichokes.

<u>Volcano Buffalo Chicken</u> – Hot sauce, chicken celery and ranch dressing.

<u>BBQ Chicken</u> – Grilled chicken, onion and bacon. I ask the waitperson to ask the chef to substitute extra chicken for the bacon.

<u>Margherita</u> – Tomato, mozzarella and basil.

<u>Mediterranean</u> – Fresh mozzarella, Kalamata olives, capers, and red onion.

Paul Mineo's Trattoria
Maryland Heights, MO

Appetizers:

Italian Meatballs – In our homemade meat sauce.

Pizza Bruschetta – Diced tomatoes, garlic, fresh basil, olive oil & mozzarella cheese.

Chicken Pesto Pizza – Olive oil, pesto, fresh tomatoes & grilled chicken.

Salads:

House Salad – Mixed greens in a balsamic vinaigrette dressing.

Caesar Salad – Traditional with homemade croutons. I ask the waitperson to ask the chef to leave off the croutons and to substitute balsamic vinaigrette dressing for the Caesar dressing.

Mineo's Special Salad – Salami, cheese, mixed greens with tomato and onion.

Insalata di Pomodoro – Tomatoes, onions & anchovies with fresh mozzarella cheese. I ask the waitperson to ask the chef to substitute extra tomato for the anchovies.

Soup of the Day – Ask server.

Entrees:

Entrees are served with mixed vegetables and roasted potatoes.

Polo Marsala – Chicken breast with mushrooms & green peppers in Marsala wine sauce.

Pollo Spiedini – Chicken, prosciutto & Fontina cheese in bread crumbs, topped with Marsala mushroom sauce. I ask the waitperson to ask the chef to leave off the prosciutto and the bread crumbs.

Pollo Carcioffi Piccata – Chicken breast with mushrooms & artichoke hearts in white wine lemon sauce.

Vitellino Alla Panna – Thin veal with artichoke hearts in a cream sauce.

Vitellino Carcioffi Piccata – Thin veal with mushrooms & artichoke hearts in white wine lemon sauce.

Vitellino Siciliano – Thin veal lightly breaded, grilled in olive oil, lemon & garlic. I ask the waitperson to ask the chef to leave off the breading.

Vitellino Di Saltimbocca – Thin veal with prosciutto ham & cheese in a white wine sage sauce. I ask the waitperson to ask the chef to leave off the prosciutto ham.

Filetto Trifolato – Beef medallions with portabella mushrooms in cabernet wine garlic sauce.

Filetto di Manzo Alla Paulo – Beef medallions with artichokes & mushrooms in port wine reduction.

Bistecca Siciliano – Prime New York Steak lightly breaded with lemon garlic sauce. I ask the waitperson to ask the chef to leave off the breading.

Pasta:

Pennate Alla Arabiata – Sautéed eggplant, mushrooms & capers in a spicy tomato sauce.

Cavetelli Con Broccoli – Shell noodles in our broccoli cream sauce with mushrooms.

Tortellini Alla Panna – Meat stuffed dumplings with mushrooms in a sherry sauce.

Mom Mineo's Famous Lasagna – Meat sauce and mix of

Italian cheeses.

<u>Risotto Milanese</u> – Peas & mushrooms with cheeses.

<u>Desserts:</u>

<u>Tiramisu</u>

<u>Chocolate Cake Overload</u>

Pelican
Albuquerque, NM

Starters:

Fresh Zucchini – Battered to order. I ask the waitperson to ask the chef to steam my zucchini.

Fresh Mushrooms – Battered to order. I ask the waitperson to ask the chef to steam my mushrooms.

Steamed Artichoke – While they last!

Steaks & Prime Rib:

We take pride in the quality of our beef, and serve USDA CHOICE Beef, properly aged and cut fresh daily, then seasoned with our own recipe of spices to complement the flavor. Served with bottomless salad bowl, choice of dressing, and one extra.

Choice Center-Cut Top Sirloin – Served on sautéed onions.

Center-Cut New York Strip – Chef Selection. Served with peppercorn gravy and onion rings. I ask the waitperson to ask the chef to put the peppercorn gravy on the side for dipping and to substitute grilled onions for the onion rings.

Choice Rib Eye

Filet Mignon – Market

Charred Rib Eye – Rubbed and marinated in our blend of spices, served with an onion ring. I ask the waitperson to ask the chef to leave off the onion ring.

Teriyaki Center-Cut Top Sirloin – Served with teriyaki sauce and a pineapple slice.

New York Strip

Prime Rib "Regular" or "Large" – Slow-roasted and served with our homemade au jus. While it lasts! I ask the waitperson to ask the chef for horseradish sauce for my prime rib.

Pelican's Signature Rib Eye – Chef's selection. Our famous prime rib grilled and served with crisp onions. I ask the waitperson to ask the chef to substitute sautéed or grilled onions for the crisp onions.

Ranchero Top Sirloin – Roasted green chili and melted Jack and cheddar cheeses.

Combinations:

Vegetarian Platter – A combination of sautéed asparagus and mushrooms and your choice of side. I order steamed vegetables for my side.

All steak combos come with our top sirloin. Ask your server about upgrading to any steak of your choice.

Chicken:

Grilled Chicken – With roasted garlic and mushrooms.

Hawaiian Chicken – Served with teriyaki sauce and a pineapple slice.

Chicken Ranchero – Roasted green chili and melted Jack and cheddar cheeses.

Baked Blackened Chicken Linguini – Chef's Selection. Served with Alfredo sauce. I eat this dish on a reward night.

Soups & Salads:

Pelican's Bottomless Salad Bowl

Caesar Salad – I ask the waitperson to ask the chef to substitute bleu cheese dressing for the Caesar dressing and to leave off the croutons.

Grilled Caesar With Chicken – I ask the waitperson to ask

the chef to substitute bleu cheese dressing for the Caesar dressing and to leave off the croutons.

Extras:

Sautéed Mushrooms

Sautéed Asparagus

Steamed Vegetables

Burgers:

Mushroom and Swiss Burger – Served with fries. I ask the waitperson to ask the chef to substitute a vegetable for the fries.

Green Chili and Cheddar – Served with fries. I ask the waitperson to ask the chef to substitute a vegetable for the fries.

Bleu Cheese and Fried Red Onion – Served with fries. I ask the waitperson to ask the chef to substitute a vegetable for the fries and to substitute red onion for the fried red onion.

Plain Jane – Served with fries. I ask the waitperson to ask the chef to substitute a vegetable for the fries.

Additional Toppings – Monterey Jack, Cheddar, Bleu Cheese Crumbles, Sautéed Mushrooms, Sautéed Onions, Green Chili.

Early Bird:

Reduced portions served from 5:00 'til 6:30 daily. Served with our bottomless salad bowl and your choice of a side.

Teriyaki Center-Cut Top Sirloin – Top sirloin grilled with vegetables and teriyaki sauce.

Hawaiian Chicken – Served with teriyaki sauce and a pineapple slice.

<u>Desserts:</u>

<u>Chocolate Mousse Cake</u>

<u>Cheesecake</u>

The Pie Pantry
Belleville, IL
Family Restaurant

Appetizers:

Quesadillas – Choice of veggie, steak, or cheese with salsa and sour cream.

Scrumptious Salads:

Dressings: Italian, French, Blue Cheese, Ranch, or Raspberry Vinaigrette.

Ellie's Chicken Salad Platter – Made with pineapple, pecans, celery, and red peppers, served with fresh fruit and home-made Hawaiian bread.

Spinach Salad – With egg, mushrooms, sliced almonds and warm bacon dressing. Grilled chicken is available for an additional charge. I ask the waitperson to ask the chef to substitute blue cheese dressing for the bacon dressing.

Caesar Salad – Romaine lettuce, eggs, green onions, carrots and diced bacon tossed with parmesan cheese and our special dressing. Chicken is available for an additional charge. I ask the waitperson to ask the chef to substitute extra romaine for the bacon and to substitute blue cheese dressing for the special dressing.

Chef Salad – Crisp lettuce, tomato, fresh mushrooms, cheddar cheese, chopped egg, ham, turkey and croutons with your choice of dressing. I ask the waitperson to ask the chef to substitute extra turkey for the ham and to substitute extra tomato for the croutons.

Super Chef Salad – Add a scoop of chicken salad to our regular chef salad.

<u>Fresh Garden Salad</u> – Crisp lettuce, tomato, green onions and cheese served with your choice of dressing.

Savory Soups:

Available daily: Chili, French Onion, and Soup Du Jour. On the French Onion soup I ask the waitperson to ask the chef to leave off all bread and croutons.

Combos and Bonanzas:

<u>Soup and Salad Combo</u> – A cup of soup with your choice of a Garden, Spinach, or Caesar Salad, with a home-made pantry roll.

<u>Soup and Sandwich Combo</u> – A cup of soup with one half of these sandwiches: Chicken Salad or Pantry Chicken served with your choice of a side.

<u>Bonanza</u> – A cup of soup with choice of salad and half sandwich as listed above.

Scrumptious Sandwiches:

Served with fresh fruit.

<u>Chicken Salad Sandwich</u> – A Pie Pantry original. Made with almonds, celery and chopped eggs and served on toasted raisin bread.

<u>Ellie's Chicken Salad Sandwich</u> – Made with pineapple, celery, red peppers and pecans, served on toasted raisin bread.

<u>Rueben</u> – Corned beef, Swiss cheese, sauerkraut and 1000 Island Dressing on toasted marble rye. I ask the waitperson to ask the chef to substitute yellow mustard for the 1000 Island Dressing.

<u>Grilled Chicken Breast Sandwich</u> – Juicy plump grilled chicken breast served with lettuce and tomato on a pantry roll.

Burgers:

Burger – 6 ounces of seasoned meat with lettuce, tomato, onions and pickle served on a grilled pantry roll. Cheese is available for an additional charge.

Gourmet Burger – Topped with onions, mushrooms, bacon, cheddar and Swiss cheese. I ask the waitperson to ask the chef to substitute extra onions for the bacon.

Wonderful Wraps:

Turkey Club Wrap – Turkey, bacon, cheddar cheese, lettuce, tomato and ranch dressing rolled up in a warm flour tortilla. I ask the waitperson to ask the chef to substitute extra turkey for the bacon.

Chicken Caesar Wrap – A Caesar salad with grilled chicken breast wrapped in a warm flour tortilla. I ask the waitperson to ask the chef to substitute blue cheese dressing for the Caesar dressing on the salad.

For the Little Ones:

10 and under please.

Burger Plate served with fries. I ask the waitperson to ask the chef to substitute lettuce and tomatoes for the fries.

Chicken Strip Plate served with fries. I ask the waitperson to ask the chef to substitute grilled chicken or the chicken strips and to substitute lettuce and tomatoes for the fries.

Pie Pantry Pies:

Apple

Peach

Custard

Rhubarb

Specialty Pies:

Pecan Cheesecake

Turtle Cheesecake

Chocolate Chip Cheesecake

Chocolate Chip Pecan

French Silk

Black Forest

Pecan

Special Order and Seasonal Pies:

Strawberry

Strawberry-Rhubarb

Ponderosa Steakhouse:
International Chain Restaurant

All You Can Eat Buffet – Salads, vegetables, pasta, desserts.
½ Pound Sirloin – USDA Choice.
10 oz. Top Sirloin – Center cut.
10 oz. Ribeye
1 lb. T-Bone
Sirloin Tips
Chicken Monterey or Grilled Chicken
Three Steak Medallions
Chopped Steak
½ Pound Cheeseburger or Grilled Chicken Sandwich
Senior Lunch Buffet
Senior Dinner Buffet

Pueblo Harvest Café & Bakery
Indian Pueblo Cultural Center
Albuquerque, NM

Served 11am to Close. The Pueblo Harvest Café proudly serves locally grown and harvested ingredients!

Appetizers:

I eat appetizers on a reward day.

Cheese Quesadilla – A layer of shredded cheddar/Jack cheese sandwiched in a homemade tortilla. For an additional charge you can add sautéed vegetables, chicken, or beef. Served with fresh homemade salsa and sour cream.

Nachos – Tri-color tortilla chips, served with melted cheddar/Jack cheese, sliced jalapenos, freshly diced tomatoes, black olives and lettuce. For an additional charge you can add grilled chicken or ground buffalo, lamb, or ground beef. Served with salsa and sour cream.

Stews:

All stews are gluten free.

Green Chili Stew

Mutton Stew

Salads:

Dressings: Ranch, House Vinaigrette, Bleu Cheese, and Red Chili Vinaigrette. All dressings are gluten free. I eat fry bread on a reward day.

Cochiti Cob Salad – Spring mix topped with roasted turkey, bacon, diced tomato, boiled egg, sliced avocado, black olives, roasted corn, and topped with queso fresco. I ask the waitperson to ask the chef to substitute extra spring mix and diced tomatoes for the bacon and avocado.

Indian Taco Salad – Carne adovada atop mixed greens, roasted corn, freshly diced tomatoes, finished with queso fresco. Served on fry bread. I ask the waitperson to ask the chef to substitute ground beef or buffalo for the carne adovada.

North Valley "Greek" Salad – Spring mix, artichoke hearts, sliced avocado, diced tomato, shaved red onions, black olives, and local queso fresco. I ask the waitperson to ask the chef to substitute extra tomatoes for the avocado.

Harvest House Salad – Chopped romaine lettuce topped with oven bread croutons, dried cranberries, fresh herbs, sliced apples, and queso fresco. I ask the waitperson to ask the chef to substitute extra romaine lettuce for the oven bread croutons.

Pueblo Caesar Salad with Grilled Chicken – Chopped romaine lettuce topped with oven bread croutons, black pepper/pinon/parmesan crumbles, fried capers and shaved red onions. I ask the waitperson to ask the chef to substitute extra romaine lettuce for the oven bread croutons and to substitute bleu cheese dressing for the Caesar dressing.

Sandwiches & Burgers:

All sandwiches are served with your choice of fruit salad or calabacitas (mixed vegetables).

Albuquerque Turkey – Oven roasted turkey breast served with diced Bueno ® green chili, grilled tomatoes and pepper Jack cheese on oven bread.

San Felipe Chicken Sandwich – Grilled chicken breast served on a Kaiser roll with garlic herb mayo, lettuce, and tomato.

San Ildefonso Sandwich – Grilled Portobello mushroom topped with avocado, sliced tomatoes, grilled onions, and finished with melted pepper Jack cheese and red chili vinaigrette. I ask the waitperson to ask the chef to substitute extra tomatoes for the avocado.

Santa Fe Burger – All ground beef patty served with mushrooms, avocado, and Swiss cheese. I ask the waitperson to ask the chef to substitute tomato for the avocado.

Picuris Patty Melt – All ground beef patty served with Bueno® green chili, cheddar cheese, and grilled onions on our green chili cheddar oven bread. You can substitute a buffalo patty or roasted sliced lamb for an additional charge.

BYO Burger

Choose your patty: Hand pressed beef or can substitute buffalo or lamb for an additional charge.

Choose your cheese: Swiss, cheddar or pepper Jack.

Choose your bread: Fry bread, Pueblo oven bread, homemade tortilla, or a burger bun.

Entrees:

Chicken Nambe Relleno – A large poblano chili stuffed with a savory mix of cheddar cheese and chicken, rolled in blue corn meal and topped with red chili sauce. Served with Pueblo beans and calabacitas. Ask your server for the vegetarian option. I ask the waitperson to ask the chef to substitute extra calabacitas for the Pueblo beans.

Tewa Taco (our world famous "Indian" taco) – Ground beef and Pueblo beans served on top of homemade fry bread and garnished with cheese, lettuce, tomatoes, onions and a choice of red or green chili. I ask the waitperson to ask the chef to substitute extra lettuce and tomatoes for the Pueblo beans.

A La Carte:

Side of one egg.

Side of Nambe Relleno.

Side of beef patty.

Side of chicken breast.

Side of red or green chili sauce.

Side of fruit.

Pueblo Selections:

All entrees are served with fresh oven bread and pinion butter. A Harvest House Salad can be added for an additional charge.

Bison Short Ribs – Braised in red wine until falling off the bone, served with ancho chili, demi-glace, and the chef selected sides of the day.

Slow Roasted 10 oz. Prime Rib Au Jus – Served with horseradish sauce, green chili mashed potatoes, and sautéed vegetables. I ask the waitperson to ask the chef to substitute extra vegetables for the mashed potatoes.

Rack of New Mexico Lamb – Locally raised lamb crusted in sunflower seeds and served with a mint pesto and smoked tomato demi-glace.

Desserts:

Ohkay Owingeh Oven Bread Pudding – With caramel sauce.

Rainforest Café
International Chain Restaurant

Appetizers:

Rainforest Pita Quesadillas – A new twist on an old favorite! Grilled chicken, roasted peppers, caramelized onions and melted cheese on grilled pita bread. Served with fresh pico de gallo and sour cream.

Chile Con Queso – Creamy melted cheese with tomatoes, onions and green chile peppers served with tri-colored tortilla chips. With seasoned ground beef added.

Lava Nachos – A hot favorite from south of the border! Crispy tri-colored tortilla chips topped with seasoned ground beef, peppers, onions, black beans, corn and cheddar cheese. Garnished with green onions, sour cream and pico de gallo. I ask the waitperson to ask the chef to substitute extra cheddar cheese and green onions for the black beans and corn.

Spinach & Artichoke Dip – Creamy spinach, tender artichokes, parmesan and cream cheese, topped with pico de gallo and served with warm crispy tri-colored tortilla chips.

Brave New World Flatbread – Flatbread topped with charbroiled, hand-pulled chicken breast, our Smokin' Mojo BBQ sauce, mozzarella cheese and chopped cilantro.

Soups & Salads:

Tomato Basil Soup – Tomato basil soup garnished with parmesan cheese.

Paradise Chopped House Salad – Mixed greens, Roma tomatoes, carrots and cucumbers with your choice of dressing. I ask the waitperson to ask the chef to substitute extra Roma tomatoes for the cucumbers.

Big Islander Chicken Caesar Salad – A classic Caesar salad topped with grilled chicken and grated parmesan. I ask the waitperson to ask the chef to substitute blue cheese dressing for the Caesar dressing and to leave off the croutons.

Volcanic Cobb Salad – Grilled chicken breast, romaine and iceberg lettuce, crumbled blue cheese, black olives, diced tomatoes, chopped egg, carrots and bacon. Tossed in our Paradise Balsamic Vinaigrette dressing. I ask the waitperson to ask the chef to substitute extra carrots for the bacon.

Journey Combo – Pair your choice of soup with either a half-sized chicken salad sandwich or any half-sized fresh salad.

China Island Chicken Salad – Crisp greens tossed with grilled chicken breast, potato sticks, sesame seeds, carrots, rice noodles and scallions. Tossed with our China Island salad dressing. I ask the waitperson to ask the chef to substitute extra crisp greens for the potato sticks and the rice noodles.

Ozzie's Omelette – Our 3 egg omelette built with your choice of 3 of the following items: cheddar cheese, onions, mushrooms, turkey, tomatoes, black olives, roasted red peppers or spinach. Served with fresh fruit.

Tropical Island Salad – Crisp romaine and spring mix lettuce with grilled chicken, mangos, strawberries, grapes and roasted pumpkin seeds tossed in a honey lime vinaigrette dressing.

Sandwiches & Burgers:

Rainforest Burger – Our 100% beef burger topped with a fried onion ring. Served on a toasted bun with lettuce, tomato, pickles and cheese. Add sautéed mushrooms for an additional charge. I ask the waitperson to substitute raw onion for the fried onion ring.

The Beastly Burger – Two of our 100% beef burgers topped with a fried onion ring. Served on a toasted bun with lettuce, tomato, pickles and cheese. Add sautéed mushrooms for an additional charge. I ask the waitperson to substitute raw onion for the fried onion ring.

Blue Mountain Chicken Sandwich – Lemon marinated grilled chicken breasts, topped with bacon, Swiss cheese, roasted red peppers and leaf lettuce. Served on herbed Asiago ciabatta bread with our zesty Safari sauce. I ask the waitperson to ask the chef to substitute extra roasted red peppers for the bacon.

Portabella Wrap – Tomato basil wrap layered and rolled with spinach, red onions, roasted red peppers and grilled portabella mushrooms, tossed in roasted garlic balsamic dressing.

Chicken Salad Sandwich – Pulled chicken, tossed with tarragon, celery, onions, toasted almonds and mayonnaise. Served on a croissant with lettuce and tomato.

Bamba's Barbecue Wrap – Shredded beef or chicken with our Smokin' Mojo BBQ sauce, fresh cilantro, onions and mozzarella cheese wrapped in a flour tortilla. Served with mango sauce.

Rio's Rueben – A classic Reuben with corned beef, melted Swiss cheese,steamy sauerkraut and Thousand Island dressing on grilled marble rye. I ask the waitperson to ask the chef to substitute spicy mustard for the Thousand Island dressing.

Philly Cheese Steak – Traditional style cheese steak with sautéed onions and peppers, topped with melted Monterey Jack and Swiss cheeses, served with lettuce and tomatoes on a toasted hoagie roll.

Beef, Pork, & Chicken:

Hickory Chicken – Marinated and grilled boneless chicken breasts brushed with our Smokin' Mojo BBQ sauce topped with sautéed mushrooms and melted Jack cheese. Served with red skinned mashed potatoes and your choice of a side. I ask the waitperson to ask the chef to substitute a vegetable for the mashed potatoes.

Amazon Fajitas – Sizzling chicken or beef fajitas, served over grilled onions and bell peppers. Served with sour cream, fresh guacamole, lettuce, Cheddar cheese, pico de gallo, Caribbean rice, black beans and warm flour tortillas. I ask the waitperson to ask the chef to substitute extra lettuce for the guacamole and to substitute extra grilled onions and bell peppers for the rice and black beans.

Beef Chicken Combo:

Flat Iron Steak Combo – Our char-grilled flat iron steak topped with steak butter and served and served with your choice of fried shrimp, Caribbean Coconut Shrimp or with ¼ rotisserie chicken. Served with red skinned mashed potatoes and your choice of a side. I order the chicken and ask the waitperson to ask the chef to substitute a vegetable for the mashed potatoes.

Paradise Pot Roast – This will get your taste buds talking! Tender, thick-sliced pot roast and vegetables over red skinned mashed potatoes and served in its natural juices. Beef Chicken Combo. I ask the waitperson to ask the chef to substitute a vegetable for the mashed potatoes.

Rotisserie Chicken – Half of a slow-roasted chicken served with red skinned mashed potatoes and your choice of a side. I ask the waitperson to ask the chef to substitute a vegetable for the mashed potatoes.

Pasta:

Tropical Tortellini – Tri-colored cheese tortellini with sun-dried tomatoes, peas and mushrooms tossed in Alfredo sauce. Add grilled chicken for an additional charge.

Portofino Pasta – Sautéed zucchini, yellow squash, sun-dried and Roma tomatoes tossed with linguini, arugula, fresh mozzarella cheese and basil oil. Add grilled chicken for an additional charge.

<u>Rasta Pasta</u> – Grilled chicken, cavatappi pasta, walnut pesto, broccoli, red peppers and spinach tossed with garlic Alfredo sauce.

<u>Sides:</u>

<u>Seasonal Vegetables</u>

<u>Coleslaw</u>

Red Robin
International Chain Restaurant

Appetizers:

Classic Mini Wedge Salad – Topped with bleu cheese crumbles, bacon bits, onion straws, diced tomatoes and ranch dressing. I ask the waitperson to ask the chef to substitute extra tomatoes for the bacon bits and to substitute raw onion for the onion straws.

Creamy Artichoke & Spinach Dip – Cheesy and delicious. Served with celery sticks and sea salt tortilla chips.

Chili Chili™ Con Queso – Red's Chili Chili™ and creamy queso. Topped with salsa garnish and sea salt tortilla chips.

Fresh Salads:

The Red, White & Bleu – This salad is a star with cranberries, apple slices and bleu cheese. Mixed with grilled chicken and candied walnuts and tossed in a Dijon vinaigrette. Served with garlic focaccia.

Simply Grilled Chicken Salad – Our juicy grilled chicken breast, cheddar cheese, tomatoes, cucumbers and croutons on a bed of mixed greens. Served with garlic focaccia and a choice of dressing. I ask the waitperson to ask the chef to substitute extra tomatoes and mixed greens for the cucumbers and croutons.

Soup & Salad Combo – Your favorite bowl of soup served with a crisp mixed-greens house salad.

House Salad

Soups:

French Onion Soup – Say "oui" to this fresh favorite topped with melted provolone and parmesan. Served with garlic focaccia. I ask the waitperson to ask the chef to prepare my onion soup without bread or croutons.

Chicken Tortilla Soup – Hearty chicken and vegetables, topped with cheddar, sour cream and tortilla strips. I ask the waitperson to ask the chef to leave off the tortilla strips.

Red's Chili Chili – What do you do when a chili craving strikes? Order our meaty blend of beans, spices and hearty peppers quickly. Topped with cheddar, onions and tortilla strips. I ask the waitperson to ask the chef to leave off the tortilla strips.

Wraps & Sandwiches:

Wraps and sandwiches are served with Freckled Fruit Salad.

Caesar's Chicken Wrap – A natural leader, this wrap rules with sliced grilled, chicken breast, parmesan, tomatoes, romaine lettuce and Caesar dressing wrapped in a fresh spinach tortilla. I ask the waitperson to ask the chef to substitute bleu cheese dressing for the Caesar dressing.

Baja Turkey Club – It's a club with a kick. Sliced turkey breast, roasted green chile, cheddar, pepper-Jack, tomatoes & hardwood-smoked bacon on Texas toast with green chile aioli. I ask the waitperson to ask the chef to substitute extra cheddar for the bacon and to leave off the middle slice of bread.

Whiskey River BBQ Chicken Wrap – We corralled the renegade of flavors of the Southwest in a tasty spinach tortilla; grilled chicken with tangy Whiskey River BBQ Sauce, cheddar cheese, lettuce, tortilla strips and a touch of ranch. Brace for the stampede! I ask the waitperson to ask the chef to substitute extra lettuce for the tortilla strips.

BLTA Croissant – Correct pronunciation not required! You'll get enough of a mouthful with this delicious combination of turkey breast, hardwood-smoked bacon, mayo and, of course, lettuce, tomato and avocado. I ask the waitperson to ask the chef to substitute extra lettuce and tomato for the bacon and the avocado.

Fire-Grilled Burgers:

Red Robin Gourmet Cheeseburger – The one that made us famous. Featuring Red Robin's pickle relish, tomatoes, onions, lettuce, pickles, mayo and a choice of cheese.

Bleu Ribbon – A highly prized burger! Topped with tangy steak sauce, chipotle aioli, bleu cheese, lettuce, tomato and crispy onion straws. Served on an onion bun, it's the envy of the country fair. I ask the waitperson to ask the chef to substitute grilled onion for the crispy onion straws.

Chili Chili™ Cheeseburger – You might need an extra napkin. Served open face with a generous helping of Red's Chili Chili™ , cheddar cheese, chipotle aioli and diced red onions. Cleanup crew not included.

Grilled Turkey – Gobble up our deliciously seasoned turkey patty served on whole grain bun with zesty chipotle aioli, lettuce and tomatoes.

Red's Tavern Double – You'll be tasking double with two classic-size patties, melted American cheese, tomato, lettuce and Red's secret Tavern Sauce. I ask the waitperson to ask the chef to substitute Swiss or cheddar cheese for the American cheese.

Banzai – The burger of the beach bums, surfer dudes and hungry people. Glazed in teriyaki and topped with grilled pineapple, cheddar, lettuce, tomatoes and mayo for a taste wave that'll knock you off your board.

Sautéed 'Shroom – Mushrooms of the world we salute you! Topped with melted Swiss and garlic parmesan spread.

Prime Chophouse – White gloves are not required. A fire-grilled burger layered with horseradish-sautéed mushrooms, gourmet steak sauce, provolone, country Dijon and crispy onion straws on an onion bun. Good thing you aren't wearing gloves, because this could get messy. I ask the waitperson to ask the chef to substitute grilled onion for the crispy onion straws.

Whiskey River BBQ – Our smoky, tangy tribute to the Wild West. We roped together our signature Bourbon-infused Whiskey River BBQ sauce, crispy onion straws, cheddar, lettuce, tomato and mayo. See if you can hang onto it for eight seconds. I ask the waitperson to ask the chef to substitute grilled onion for the crispy onion straws.

All-American Patty Melt – Some perfection can't be messed with – like sautéed onions and Thousand Island dressing on marbled rye. But you can add to the perfection by choosing your favorite cheese. I ask the waitperson to ask the chef to substitute spicy mustard for the Thousand Island dressing.

Customize Your Order:

We make everything to order, so if you want to customize anything let us know.

Side Salad

Steamed Broccoli

Coleslaw

Freckled Fruit™ Salad

Cup of Soup

Cup of Chili Chili

Chicken Burgers:

Anything between two buns is a burger to us, even if it is made with a premium-quality whole chicken breast.

Whiskey River™ BBQ Chicken – Grilled chicken breast basted with our Bourbon-infused Whisker River™ BBQ Sauce topped with melted cheddar, crispy onion straws, lettuce, tomatoes and mayo. It's only found around these here parts. I ask the waitperson to ask the chef to substitute grilled onion for the onion straws.

Teriyaki Chicken – Channel your inner ninja with this perfectly grilled chicken breast, teriyaki, grilled pineapple, Swiss, lettuce, tomatoes and mayo.

Simply Grilled Chicken – A perfectly grilled chicken breast served on a sesame bun with lettuce, tomatoes, pickles and onions on the side with your choice of Bottomless Steak Fries™ or bottomless Freckled Fruit™ Salad. I order the fruit salad.

Bruschetta Chicken – Take a culinary trip through the Italian countryside with a perfectly grilled chicken breast topped with fresh bruschetta salsa, pesto aioli, provolone, romaine lettuce and balsamic cream on a rustic ciabatta. It's a true renaissance burger.

Entrees:

Fun without a bun.

Prime Rib Dip – Watch your table manners with this rustic combination of tender sliced prime rib with caramelized onions, horseradish sauce, provolone and au jus (which is just a fancy word for delicious). Served with coleslaw and Bottomless Steak Fries. I ask the waitperson to ask the chef to substitute a side salad for the fries.

Ensenada Chicken™ Platter – For intense Baja-style flavor, look no farther than the border of your plate. Two-fire grilled chicken breasts basted with authentic Mexican seasonings, topped with fresh salsa and creamy salsa-ranch. Served with a side salad. Or lighten up with only one chicken breast.

Red Robin's Finest Gourmet Burgers:

Over 40 years our burger expertise has led to this: Red Robin's finest. Juicy 1/2-pound Black Angus burgers handmade and flame-grilled to order, then stacked with the freshest premium toppings to create an exceptional burger experience.

Smoke & Pepper™ – Perhaps our finest burger yet. Topped with black-pepper bacon and extra-sharp cheddar on a toasted ciabatta bun with our house-made Smoke & Pepper ketchup. I ask the waitperson to ask the chef to substitute grilled onions for the black-pepper bacon.

Black & Bleu – A true knife-and-fork burger. Sautéed, blackened Portobello mushrooms, grilled onions, house-made bleu cheese sauce and bleu cheese crumbles on a toasted ciabatta bun with Dijon sauce.

Dessert:

End on a sweet note.

Gooey Chocolate Brownie Cake – Indulgent chocolate brownie cake and hot fudge topped with vanilla ice cream and served with sweet strawberries and berry sauce.

River Grill
Bentonville, AR

Appetizers:

Charcuterie Board – Chef's selection of meats and cheeses, marinated olives, grapes and fried capers. Served with crostini. I ask the waitperson to ask the chef to substitute extra olives for the grapes.

Soup and Salads:

Cup/Bowl of Soup du Jour

River Grill Chopped Salad – Iceburg and butter lettuce with chopped tomatoes, onions, bacon and parmesan ribbons. I ask the waitperson to ask the chef to substitute extra lettuce and tomato for the bacon.

River Mesclun Salad – Mesclun greens tossed with orange-poppy dressing and finished with gorgonzola, sliced granny apples, walnut brittle and sweet potato frites. I ask the waitperson to ask the chef to substitute extra apples for the sweet potato frites.

Spinach and Arugula Salad – Delicately tossed spinach and arugula in sherry-Dijon vinaigrette. Finished with Stilton blue cheese, bacon and pine nuts. I ask the waitperson to ask the chef to substitute extra pine nuts for the bacon.

Side Dishes:

Sautéed Spinach with Bacon – I ask the waitperson to ask the chef to leave off the bacon.

Seasonal Vegetables

Fresh Asparagus with Parmesan and Pine Nuts

Shitake and Crimini mushrooms in Burgundy Beef Reduction

Steaks and Chops:

Steak Tournedos – Served on truffled potato crostini with asparagus finished with gorgonzola demi-glace. I ask the waitperson to ask the chef to substitute extra asparagus for the potato crostini.

Master Cut 16 oz. Ribeye USDA Prime

Ribeye 12 oz. USDA Prime

Beef Tenderloin Filet 10 oz.

Beef Tenderloin Filet 7 oz.

New York Strip 14 oz.

Bison Tenderloin – 8 oz. bison tenderloin with a port wine demi-glace.

Date Night Menu:

First Course – Cuban black bean salad.

Second Course – Pesto Caprese – Sliced tomatoes and fresh mozzarella over basil pesto.

Third Course – N.Y. Strip Steak served with roasted garlic gournay whipped potatoes finished with honey mustard balsamic glaze. I ask the waitperson to ask the chef to substitute the fresh asparagus with parmesan and pine nuts for the whipped potatoes.

Fourth Course – Tiramisu

Ruby Tuesday
International Chain Restaurant

Appetizers:

Queso and Chips

Chicken Quesadillas

Three-Cheese Spinach Dip and Chips

Salad Bar:

Fresh Steamed Broccoli

Romaine Lettuce

Spring Mix

Raw Red Onion Rings

Fresh Mushrooms

Sunflower Kernels

Diced Eggs

Shredded Jack, Parmesan and Cheddar Cheese

Coleslaw

Sliced Raw Tomatoes

Diced Raw Tomatoes

Salad Bar with No Fat Dressing – Romaine, broccoli, Parmesan cheese, tomatoes, peppers, onions, eggs and fat-free ranch dressing.

Salad Bar with Regular Dressing – Romaine, Jack and cheddar cheeses, tomatoes, bacon, onions and ranch dressing. I leave off the bacon.

Salads:

Buffalo Chicken Salad

Salad Dressing:

Light Ranch Dressing – A dip for veggies.

Ranch Dressing – For side salad.

Vinaigrette Dressing – For side salads.

Blue Cheese Dressing – Dip for buffalo wings and side salads.

Soups:

White Chicken Chili

Baked French Onion Soup – I ask the waitperson to ask the chef to prepare my soup without any croutons or bread.

Cooked Vegetables:

Sautéed Fresh Zucchini

Fajita Vegetables – Onions and peppers.

Meat Dishes:

Fajitas Steak Meat Alone – Grilled top sirloin steak beef tips.

Ribeye Steak – Seasoned 12 oz. Ribeye steak.

Top Sirloin Steak – Seasoned 7 oz. or 9 oz. top sirloin.

Top Sirloin Steak Meal – Seasoned 7 oz. top sirloin with steak butter and steamed broccoli and low carb mashed creamy cauliflower. I ask the waitperson to ask the chef to substitute a side salad for the cauliflower.

Petite Sirloin Steak

Fajitas Chicken Meat Alone – Grilled Cajun chicken breast.

Grilled Cajun Chicken Alone – Grilled chicken breast only.

Cajun Chicken Meal – Grilled chicken breast and steamed broccoli and low carb mashed creamy cauliflower. I ask the waitperson to ask the chef to substitute a side salad for the cauliflower.

Hamburger Patty – 8 oz. plain.

Bacon Cheeseburger – Served with your choice of fries or a spring mix salad. I order the salad and ask the waitperson to ask the chef to substitute an extra slice of cheese for the bacon.

Wraps:

Turkey Wrap – No side, sliced turkey, spring mix, tomato, and Dijon mustard sauce wrapped in a whole wheat tortilla.

Spicy Chicken Wrap – No side, Cajun chicken, spring mix, cheese and creamy Dijon mustard sauce wrapped in a whole wheat tortilla.

Sadie's
Albuquerque, NM

Appetizers:

Chilie Con Queso – Served hot with fresh tostadas. I ask the waitperson to ask the chef to leave off the guacamole. I eat this appetizer on a reward night.

Shredded Beef Brisket

Chicken or Beef Taquitos – Served with salsa. Available with chilie con queso for an additional charge. I eat this appetizer on a reward night.

Dinners:

Our chilie is HOT, served on top or on the side. Choose between our red or green (made with beef), or our vegetarian green. Every dinner is topped with cheddar, lettuce, tomato, and onion.

Sadie's Enchiladas – Two soft corn tortillas stacked or rolled, served with beans. Served with Billy's spicy ground beef, chicken, or brisket. I ask the waitperson to ask the chef to substitute extra lettuce and tomato for the beans and leave off one corn tortilla.

Shredded Beef Brisket – Lean, slow cooked beef brisket. Served with frijoles and papitas, with or without chilie. I ask the waitperson to ask the chef to substitute extra lettuce and tomatoes for the frijoles and papitas.

Sadie's Burrito – A large warm flour tortilla wraps around your choice of Sadie's original grilled ground beef patty, Billy's spicy ground beef, chicken or shredded beef brisket. Served with frijoles and papitas. I ask the waitperson to ask the chef to substitute extra lettuce and tomato for the frijoles and papitas.

A La Carte:

Burrito – Served with Billy's spicy ground beef, chicken, Sadie's original lean ground beef patty, or shredded beef brisket.

Taco – with refried beans. Billy's spicy ground beef, chicken, Sadie's original lean ground beef patty, or shredded beef brisket. I ask the waitperson to ask the chef to substitute extra lettuce and tomatoes for the refried beans.

Sadie's Chef Salad – Crisp iceberg lettuce topped with fresh grated cheddar, tomato, onion, avocado, hardboiled egg and with your choice of ham or chicken. Served with Sadie's House Dressing comprised of lemon, oil, garlic and a special blend of seasonings or Green Chilie Ranch. I order the salad with the chicken and Sadie's House Dressing. I ask the waitperson to ask the chef to substitute extra tomato for the avocado.

Bowl of Chilie – Your choice of chilie served with or without beans and a flour tortilla. I order the chilie without beans.

Sadie's Original Creations:

Roberto's Special – Grilled hamburger steak generously covered with Sadie's chilie con queso, frijoles and papitas and smothered in your choice of chilie. I eat this on a reward night.

Sloppy Jose – A small mountain of Billy's spicy ground beef served on an open faced bun swimming in your choice of chilie. Served with a thick slice of French bread. I ask the waitperson to ask the chef to leave off the French bread.

Burgers:

The burger that put Sadie's on the map! Served with potato chips and your choice of thick French bread, traditional bun, flour tortilla or sopaipillas. Served with cheese or chilie. I order the bun and ask the waitperson to ask the chef to serve it open-faced, without the top bun and to substitute extra tomato for the potato chips.

Taco Burger – Served on a large corn tortilla with cheddar, lettuce, tomato, onion, and your choice of chilie on the side. Served with fries. I ask the waitperson to ask the chef to substitute extra lettuce and tomato for the fries.

Billy's Bondo Burger – Served with gaucamole and chilie con queso, grilled onions and topped with lettuce and tomato on French bread with fries. I ask the waitperson to ask the chef to substitute extra grilled onions for the gaucamole and the fries and to serve the burger open-faced, without the top slice of French bread.

From the Grill:

Upon request these dinners are smothered with your choice of chilie, served with your choice of garlic toast, sopaipillas or buttered tortillas and include a dinner salad with house dressing comprised of lemon, oil, garlic and a special blend of seasonings or Sadie's Green Chilie Ranch Dressing. On all dinners I order the house dressing and ask the waitperson to ask the chef to leave off the garlic toast, butter tortillas, and sopaipillas. I eat these dishes on a reward night.

Brian's Favorite Rib Eye Steak – Brian's personal favorite; a 12 oz. boneless lean trimmed rib eye steak charbroiled to perfection. Surrounded by frijoles and papitas. With your choice of chilie relleno, tamale, or cheese enchilada. I order the tamale. I ask the waitperson to ask the chef to substitute a small salad for the frijoles and papitas.

Sadie's Super Combination Plates – Can't decide? Sample our best! All combo plates are served with frijoles and papitas and smothered in your choice of chilie. Choose from any of the following: rolled enchilada (beef, chicken, or cheese), tamale, taco (bean, beef, chicken, guaco, guaco beef, and guaco chicken) chili relleno, a side of chilie con queso, side of guacamole, salad, chalupa (bean, beef, or chicken) or carne adovada rib. I order beef and chicken tacos and the salad. I ask the waitperson to ask the chef to substitute chilie con queso for the frijoles and papitas.

The Lighter Side:

Toni's Taco Salad – Beef or chicken served inside a flour or corn tortilla bowl with a generous portion of crisp iceberg lettuce and served with refried beans, cheddar cheese, tomato, onion, and avocado. I ask the waitperson to ask the chef to substitute extra salad mix for the refried beans and avocado.

Amanda's Mixed Green Salad – Served with a generous portion of fresh mixed greens, blue cheese crumbles, dried cranberry, pinion nuts and red chilie vinaigrette dressing. For an additional charge you can add steak or grilled chicken.

Side Orders:

Dinner Salad

Sadie's Salad

Side of Chilie Con Queso

Desserts:

Classic Cheesecake

Strawberry Cheese Cake

Ben & Jerry's® Ice Cream – Cherry Garcia, Chocolate Chip Cookie Dough, Chocolate and Fudge Brownie.

Ice Cream Sandwich

Santa Fe Grille
Santa Rosa, NM

Sandwiches:

Grilled Turkey

Veggie Sandwich

Buffalo Chicken Melt

Philly Melt

French Dip

Mexican Food:

Fajitas

Tacos

Dinners:

Chicken Stir Fry

Pot Roast

Meat Loaf

Steaks:

Rib Eye Steak

Prime Rib Steak

Ground Round Steak

Salads:

Tortilla Bowls – Chicken or Taco. I do not eat the tortilla bowl.

Asian Salad

Chef Salad

Desserts:

Banana Split

Chocolate Cake

Schneithorst
Ladue, MO

Appetizers [Vorspeisen]:

Red Pepper Hummus – Served with grilled pita bread and Kalamata olives. I do not eat the pita bread.

Soups & Salads [Salate & Suppen]:

Dressings: Ranch, Bleu Cheese, Balsamic, Mustard Vinaigrette, and Italian. Add chicken to your dinner or salad for an additional charge.

Dinner Salad – Mixed greens with grape tomatoes, sliced red onions, shredded Parmesan cheese and croutons. I ask the waitperson to ask the chef to leave off the croutons.

Organic Spinach Salad – Baby spinach, sliced mushrooms, grape tomatoes, shredded cheddar cheese, and candied walnuts tossed in balsamic dressing.

Wedge Salad – A crisp iceberg wedge with bacon, bleu cheese crumbles, tomatoes, red onions and bleu cheese dressing. I ask the waitperson to ask the chef to substitute extra tomatoes for the bacon.

Cobb Salad – Mixed greens with chopped bacon, ham, turkey, tomatoes, Kalamata olives, bleu cheese crumbles and diced egg. I ask the waitperson to ask the chef to substitute extra tomatoes and mixed greens for the chopped bacon and ham.

Sandwich & Soup or Salad Combo – Your choice of half a Turkey Sandwich or Chicken Salad Sandwich paired with a cup of soup or a dinner salad.

11 Vegetable Soup, Soup of the Day, or Red Chili Colorado

Burgers & Sandwiches:

Served with steak fries. I ask the waitperson to substitute a vegetable for the fries. For an additional charge Swiss, Monterey Jack, Pepper Jack, Cheddar or creamy Roquefort can be added.

Classic Burger – An 8 ounce patty served on a Kaiser bun with lettuce, tomatoes, onions and choice of a side.

Chicken Breast Sandwich – Marinated 8 ounce chicken breast grilled and served with lettuce, tomatoes, and onions on your choice of bread. Served with a side.

Bison Burger – Range-fed bison patty from Sayerbrook Farm, MO with your choice of bun and a side.

Chicken Salad – Served on a croissant with lettuce and tomatoes.

Dinner Entrees [Abendessen Gerichte]:

Side options for dinner entrees include the following: coleslaw, green beans, vegetable of the day, sweet & sour red cabbage, steamed broccoli and walnut carrot slaw. Asparagus is available for an additional charge.

Roasted Turkey & Dressing – In haus roasted turkey with dressing, mashed potatoes, green beans and gravy. I ask the waitperson to ask the chef to leave off the gravy and to substitute coleslaw for the dressing and steamed broccoli for the potatoes.

Chicken Vienna – Sautéed chicken breast with Gruyere cheese wrapped in black forest ham. Served with rice and asparagus accompanied with creamy paprika sauce. I ask the waitperson to ask the chef to leave off the ham and to substitute the vegetable of the day for the rice.

Beef Tournedos – Beef medallions sautéed to your liking and served with mushroom, onion, and bleu cheese demi-glace.

Served with your choice of starch and vegetable. I order the green beans and steamed broccoli.

Traditional Sauerbraten – Beef flank steak marinated for 48 hours in red wine vinegar and spices then slow-braised until fork tender. Served with haus spatzle, red cabbage, and sauerbraten gravy. I ask the wait person to ask the chef to substitute the vegetable of the day for the haus spatzle.

 Filet Mignon – An 8 ounce Certified Angus beef filet grilled to your liking and served with mashed potatoes and the vegetable du jour. I ask the waitperson to ask the chef to substitute green beans for the potatoes.

Wiener Schnitzel – Medallions of tender veal pounded thin, pan-fried and topped with a lemon caper sauce. Served with haus spatzle and red cabbage. I ask the waitperson to ask the chef to substitute the walnut carrot slaw for the haus spatzle.

Schneithorst Stroganoff – Egg noodles covered in our rich mushroom beef ragout sauce and topped with sour cream. I eat stroganoff on a reward day.

Sweets [Nachtische]:

Haus-Made Apple Strudel

Sugar-Free Apple or Cherry Pie

Banana Nut and Raisin Bread Pudding – Served with caramel sauce.

Sizzler
International Chain Restaurant

Sizzlin' Specials:

New! Endless Salad Bar Options

Roasted Rainbow Carrot Salad – Romaine, Swiss chard and roasted rainbow carrots tossed with lemon rosemary vinaigrette, topped with feta cheese.

Spiced Pumpkin Soup – Creamy pumpkin soup spiced with fresh ginger and coriander.

Hand-cut Steaks:

Fresh, USDA Choice steaks hand-cut daily. Includes choice of a side.

Tri-Tip Sirloin 8 oz. – Our signature steak. Perfectly seasoned and full of flavor.

New York Strip 12 oz. – Prized for flavor and tenderness.

Ribeye 14 oz. – Well-marbled, tender and delicious.

Burgundy Mushroom Sirloin Tips – Tri-tip served in rich wine sauce served over rice. I ask the waitperson to ask the chef to substitute a vegetable for the rice.

Steak Combos:

Featuring our Tri-tip sirloin steak 6 oz.

Steak & Chicken – Malibu or New! Italian herb.

Ribs & Chicken:

Includes a choice of a side.

New Italian Herb Chicken – 7 oz. citrus marinated chicken

breast served with fresh sautéed spinach.

Endless Salad Bar:

Endless salads, soups, hot appetizers & desserts.

Burgers & Sandwiches:

Includes choice of a side.

Double Mega Bacon Cheeseburger – Two fresh ground beef patties piled high with bacon and cheese. I ask the waitperson to ask the chef to substitute lettuce and tomato for the bacon.

Grilled Chicken Club – 7 oz. chicken breast topped with bacon and Swiss cheese. I ask the waitperson to ask the chef to substitute lettuce and tomato for the bacon and to leave off the center slice of bread.

Classic 1/3 Pound Burger – Prepared with 100% fresh ground beef. Cheese and additional patties extra.

Lunch Specials:

Same as above only smaller portions.

Sides:

Vegetable Medley

New! Sautéed Spinach

New! Seasonal Vegetable

Surf & Sirloin
Des Peres, MO

A La Carte:

Beef Vegetable Soup

Soup Du Jour

Premium Side Dish Substitutions:

Creamed or Sautéed Spinach

Fresh Asparagus

Spinach Salad

Choice of Dressings Include:

Ranch, Italian, Blue Cheese, Blue or Feta Cheese crumbles.

Sirloin:

Entrees include a baked potato and fresh vegetable of the day. For an additional charge you can add a small side salad, Greek, or Caesar salad with dinner. On all entrees I ask the waitperson to ask the chef to substitute an extra vegetable for the baked potato.

Filet Mignon – With Béarnaise sauce.

Pepperloin – With Cognac peppercorn sauce.

Tenderloin Kabob with Rice – Tenderloin, onions, peppers, mushrooms, veal stock & Burgundy wine. I ask the waitperson to substitute asparagus for the rice.

Chateaubriand Bouquetiere – 16 oz. center cut tenderloin served with a bouquet of fresh vegetables. (Prepared table side.) For 2.

New York Strip – 14 oz.

Porterhouse – 22 oz.

Rib Eye – 16 oz.

 Flintstone Steak – Bone-in, dry-aged rib eye. 26-37 oz.

Colorado Rack of Lamb – (Greek Style)

Eclectic:

Chicken Chardonnay – Mushrooms, lemon, Chardonnay cream reduction.

Chicken Marsala – Mushrooms in a Marsala wine sauce.

Grilled Breast of Chicken – Sweet peppers in balsamic vinegar.

Veal Piccata – Capers, mushrooms, lemon, butter & Chardonnay wine & pasta Alfredo. I ask the waitperson to substitute fresh asparagus for the pasta Alfredo.

Vegetarian – (Chef's Creation).

Desserts:

Baklava

Crème Brulee

The Tea Room at Relics
Relics Antiques Mall
Springfield, MO

Entrees:

Relics Quiche Florentine – A rich blend of cream, eggs and Swiss and parmesan cheeses accents fresh baby spinach with mushrooms in our unique, flaky individual pie crust. Served with a garden salad. I do not eat the pie crust.

Chicken Breast with Long and Wild Rice – Grilled chicken breast drizzled with our flavorful sweet but tangy orange mustard. Served with a wild rice blend of walnuts, spinach and orange segments and fresh butter sautéed green beans. I eat the rice on a reward day. On non-reward days I ask the waitperson to ask the chef to substitute extra green beans for the rice.

Soup of the day – A delicious concoction using seasonal fresh ingredients. Served with a seasoned English muffin half and a garden salad.

Sandwiches:

All sandwiches are served with multi-grain sun chips. For an additional charge you can substitute a side salad, cup of soup, or fruit. Any half sandwich can be had with soup or salad. With all sandwiches, I substitute a side salad for the sun chips.

Chicken Waldorf – Seasoned chicken breast, fresh grapes, apples, celery, red onion, dried cranberries, and English walnuts blended with creamy tarragon mayo on a freshly baked croissant.

Roasted Turkey and Baby Swiss Cheese – Oven roasted turkey breast topped with leafy greens, tomatoes, and served on whole wheat bread with herby basil mayo.

Slow Roasted Beef – (served hot) Freshly baked, tender, thin sliced roast-beef with sautéed onions on our fresh baked soft baguette topped with horseradish cheese sauce.

Rubenesque – (served hot) Thinly sliced corned beef using only the most tender portions, crowned with tart freshly sautéed cabbage covered in creamy Swiss cheese sauce. Served with our own Thousand Island dressing served on the side. I ask the waitperson to ask the chef to substitute mustard for the Thousand Island dressing.

Salads:

Served with our freshly baked garlic crostini's. You can add chicken, turkey, or beef to any salad for an additional charge.

Caesar – Garden fresh romaine lettuce, shredded parmesan cheese, sliced eggs, green olives and grape tomatoes with a classic creamy Caesar dressing. I ask the waitperson to ask the chef to substitute bleu cheese for the Caesar dressing.

Mosaic – Green leafy baby spinach and romaine lettuce filled with avocado, zucchini, bell peppers, grape tomatoes, and carrots covered with homemade dill dressing. I ask the waitperson to ask the chef to substitute extra tomatoes for the avocado.

Strawberry Fields – Fresh greens, strawberries, feta cheese, and English walnuts tossed with strawberry vinaigrette.

Desserts:

Hawaiian Carrot Cake – Moist cake with our own rich cream cheese frosting.

Brownie Ala Mode – Made with rich Ghirardelli chocolate and covered with vanilla bean ice cream.

Decadent Vanilla Cheese Cake – Smooth and creamy with your choice of topping: Chocolate Grenache or homemade salted caramel sauce.

T's Redneck Steakhouse
Lebanon, MO

Appetizers:

Hickory Smoked Wings – We'll put our wings against anyone's! A pie of fall-of-the-bone smoked wings served with our Redneck sauces: BBQ, teriyaki, hot mild, naked Thai chili sauce.

Salads:

All salads are served with our special croutons and your choice of homemade ranch or blue cheese dressing. Other dressings available: Raspberry Vinaigrette and Honey Mustard. I ask the waitperson to ask the chef to leave the croutons off my salad.

Blue Cheese Wedge – Iceberg wedges topped with diced tomatoes, red onions, bacon bits, blue cheese crumbles and house-made blue cheese dressing. Can be topped with chicken or steak. I ask the waitperson to ask the chef to leave off the bacon bits,

T's Classic Salad – Premium iceberg lettuce mixed with tomatoes, red onions, cucumbers, cheese and homemade croutons topped with your choice of grilled chicken, steak, or turkey. I ask the waitperson to ask the chef to substitute extra tomatoes for the cucumbers and to leave off the croutons.

T's Caesar Salad – Crisp Romaine lettuce sprinkled with grated parmesan, homemade croutons and a tangy Caesar dressing topped with chicken or steak. I ask the waitperson to ask the chef to substitute blue cheese dressing for the Caesar dressing and to leave off the croutons.

BBQ & Specials:

All specials are served with two sides unless noted.

Chicken Breast – A 6 oz. double breast prepared grilled. For an extra charge it is available smothered in sautéed mushrooms, onions, and melted Swiss cheese.

Turkey Dinner – A pile of our famous smoked turkey.

Steak & Beef

Our steaks are USDA Choice beef aged for 21 days for optimal tenderness. All steaks are served with freshly baked bread and two sides. Add sautéed mushrooms, onions or blue cheese crumbles!

Redneck 14 oz. Ribeye Cowboy Cut – A redneck special if you are a steak lover, you will love this tender steak.

Sirloin – Our 8 oz. sirloin is the top of the line for tenderness and flavor.

Hamburger Steak – An 8 oz. hamburger steak served with a choice of two sides.

KC Strip – 8 oz. or 6 oz.

T's Beef Tips – Hand-cut only from the most tender beef.

Prime Rib – Seasoned and slow-smoked. Served with horseradish sauce and au jus. Available Friday & Saturday after 4pm and all day Sunday. 8 oz. or 12 oz.

Sandwiches:

All sandwiches are served with your choice of one side.

Prime Rib Sandwich – 6 oz. of tender smoked prime rib topped with lettuce, tomatoes and red onions.

Smoked Turkey Bacon Club – Smoked turkey, bacon, American and Swiss cheese served on toasted white bread with lettuce and tomato. I ask the waitperson to ask the chef to substitute extra turkey for the bacon and extra Swiss cheese for the American cheese.

Chicken Breast – Grilled chicken breast topped with lettuce, red onions, tomatoes, and mayo.

Sides:

Cole Slaw

Steamed Veggies

Dinner Salad

Green Beans

T's Famous Redneck Burgers:

All of our redneck burgers are served with your choice of one side.

The Double Grilled Cheese Burger – Possibly the best burger you will ever have! A ½ pound beef patty stuffed in between two grilled cheese sandwiches. Served with lettuce, tomatoes, onions and pickles. I ask the waitperson to ask the chef to leave out the extra bread in the middle of the sandwich.

The Classic – Our ½ pound burger topped with lettuce, onions tomatoes and pickles. Can add cheese for an additional charge.

The Tightwad – A ¼ pound burger with lettuce, tomatoes, onions and pickles. Can add cheese for an additional charge.

Turkey Burger – A lean and juicy turkey patty topped with lettuce, tomatoes, onions and pickles.

The Double Blue Burger – A ½ pound burger stuffed with blue cheese crumbles and topped with lettuce, tomatoes, onions, pickles and blue cheese dressing.

Tony Roma's
International Chain Restaurant

World Famous Ribs & Combos:

This is the stuff legends are made of. The finest beef ribs, richly seasoned with select spices, slow-smoked to mouthwatering perfection. Basted with your choice of one of our signature sauces. TR's Original™ BBQ Sauce, Carolina Honeys™, Blue Ridge Smokies™, Makers Mark® Bourbon BBQ or Tony Roma's Red Hots™.

Beef Short Rib – Braised and grilled bone-in short rib topped with Cabernet demi-glace and fire-roasted zucchini, yellow squash, red peppers and carrots. Served with loaded mashed potatoes. I ask the waitperson to ask the chef to substitute extra fire-roasted vegetables for the mashed potatoes.

Bountiful Beef Ribs – Hearty ribs with a rich beef flavor. Glazed with TR's Original™ BBQ Sauce or your choice of another sauce.

Starters:

Steak & Wild Mushroom Flatbread – Crisp flatbread topped with grilled all-natural beef tenderloin, melted Havarti cheese, crumbled blue cheese, wild mushrooms, red peppers, chives and horseradish sauce.

Signature Steaks:

Filet Medallions – Three filet medallions with your choice of up to three gourmet toppings. Served with loaded mashed potatoes and your choice of a dinner salad or a cup of soup. I order the dinner salad and ask the waitperson to ask the chef to substitute a vegetable for the mashed potatoes.

12 oz. New York Strip – A heartier, leaner cut of beef with its own distinctive taste. Seasoned to perfection with Tony's special seasoning.

8 oz. Filet Mignon – A melt-in-your mouth lean cut of boneless beef tenderloin.

14 oz. Ribeye – Natural marbling makes this one of the richest, most flavorful steaks anywhere.

Chicken:

Grilled Chicken Spinach Stack – Two stacked all-natural chicken breasts straight from the open grill. Covered with a rich blend of four cheeses, artichoke hearts and creamy spinach. Served with rice and vegetables. I ask the waitperson to ask the chef to substitute extra vegetables for the rice.

BBQ ½ Chicken – A juicy half chicken basted in TR's Original™ BBQ Sauce and charbroiled. Served with French fries and coleslaw. I ask the waitperson to ask the chef to substitute a vegetable for the French fries.

Mojo Chicken – Seasoned grilled chicken breasts basted with Tony's citrus and brown mustard mojo sauce. Topped with our house made pineapple salsa and served with rice and vegetables. I ask the waitperson to ask the chef to substitute extra vegetables for the rice.

Salads and Soups:

Tony's Asian Salads – Fresh chopped Asian greens, red peppers, sweet Thai chili sauce, cilantro, fried wonton noodles and sesame seeds. Served with our Pan-Asian dressing and grilled chicken. I ask the waitperson to ask the chef to substitute extra red peppers for the fried wonton noodles.

Roma's Caesar Dinner Salad – Fresh romaine lettuce tossed in Caesar dressing and topped with shaved Asiago cheese and croutons. I ask the waitperson to ask the chef to substitute extra romaine lettuce for the croutons and to substitute blue cheese dressing for the Caesar dressing. Grilled chicken can be added for an additional charge.

Roma's Dinner Salad – Mixed greens, Roma tomato wedges, shaved Asiago cheese, croutons and red onion rings with your choice of dressing. I ask the waitperson to ask the chef to substitute extra tomato for the croutons.

Grilled Chicken & Fire-Roasted Vegetable Salad – A savory mix of grilled chicken, zucchini, yellow squash, carrots, red peppers and chives blended with chopped greens. Served with tomato pesto vinaigrette dressing and toasted cheddar flatbread.

Sandwiches:

Nolita Deli Panini – Thin sliced smoked turkey, Genoa salami, melted Havarti cheese, homemade Italian spiced pepperoncini and caper sauce on toasty Italian bread. I ask the waitperson to ask the chef to substitute extra smoked turkey for the salami.

Burgers:

Steakhouse Burger – A grilled 100% natural sirloin burger topped with Cabernet demi-glace, creamy Havarti cheese, rosemary bacon, lettuce, tomato and pickles. I ask the waitperson to ask the chef to substitute extra lettuce and tomato for the bacon.

Roma Burger – Our classic all-beef burger loaded with cheddar cheese, shredded lettuce, tomato slices, red onion and pickles.

Bistro Burger – A juicy burger topped with caramelized onions, Asiago cheese, tomato pesto and fresh mozzarella on a bakery-style bun with lettuce, pickles and a sun-dried tomato pesto sauce.

<u>Desserts:</u>

Mini desserts. The perfect size, the perfect finish.

<u>Raspberry Brownie Royale</u>

<u>Red Velvet Cake</u>

<u>Golden Apple Tart</u>

Tucano's Brazilian Grill
Chain Restaurant

Full Churrasco:

Includes assorted breads, fried bananas, unlimited Salad Festival®, an the full Churrasco Selections.

Churrasco Entrée Selections – These are some of the items brought directly to you from our wood-fired grill and carved directly onto your plate. Selections change from day to day and between lunch and dinner, but you are sure to find your favorite.

Beef:

Picanha – Top Sirloin

Fraldinha – Beef Tender

Picalho – Garlic Parmesan Beef

Assado – Marinated Beef Brisket

Carne Marinada

File Mignon com Bacon – Bacon wrapped filet mignon. I ask the waitperson to ask the chef to prepare my filet without bacon.

Poultry:

Peru – Turkey wrapped in bacon. I ask the waitperson to ask the chef to prepare my turkey without bacon.

Desserts:

Tucanos menu desserts are all made from scratch in our kitchen, using only the finest ingredients.

<u>Crème Brulee</u> – A time-honored favorite made with our special Brazilian crafting.

<u>Pudim De Leite</u> – Our Brazilian flan, richer and creamier than a traditional flan.

<u>Torre Chocolate</u> – A decadent tower of rich chocolate cake, covered in chocolate shavings, drizzled with a vanilla crème sauce and surrounded with whipped cream.

The Yellow Cactus
Floyds Knobs, IN

Starters:

Queso – Try one of our signature quesos! Chile con queso, queso picante or queso con spinach.

Nachos – Beef & chicken nachos or fajita nachos (choice of chicken or beef).

Soup & Salad:

Fajita Salad – Your choice of chicken or beef strips, peppers, onions, lettuce, tomatoes, shredded cheese and sour cream layered inside a crispy flour shell. I do not eat the crispy flour shell.

Charbroiled Chicken Salad – Grilled chicken on top of lettuce with tomatoes, onions, peppers, melted cheese, croutons and bacon bits. I ask the waitperson to ask the chef to substitute extra lettuce and tomatoes for the croutons and bacon bits.

Taco Salad – Crispy flour shell with beef or chicken, beans, lettuce, tomatoes and cheese. I do not eat the crispy flour shell.

House Salad – One trip to our salad bar.

Tortilla Soup – I ask the waitperson to ask the chef to leave off the tortilla strips.

Sandwiches:

Grilled Chicken

Fajita Sandwich

Steak Sandwich

Charbroiled Chicken Sandwich

Hamburger – Half pound.

Fajitas:

Cactus Fajita – Tender beef, chicken and chorizo cooked with onions, peppers, tomato, rice and beans served with cheese, lettuce, sour cream and tortillas. I ask the waitperson to ask the chef to substitute extra peppers and onions for the rice chorizo and beans.

Naked Fajitas – Choice of chicken or beef grilled with tomato.

Steak House Selections:

All steaks are USDA grade Choice or higher and are served with a choice of two sides. Sides: house salad, baked potato, or baked beans.

Cactus Sirloin – 6oz. or 10oz.

Cactus Ribeye – 8oz. or 12oz.

Cactus T-Bone – 16oz.

Mexican Steak Choices:

8os. Jalisco Steak – Ribeye steak sautéed with peppers, onions, and guacamole salad. Served with rice, beans and tortillas. I ask the waitperson to ask the chef to substitute a house salad for the guacamole and rice.

8oz. Steak Ranchero – Grilled Ribeye steak served with rice, beans, guacamole salad and tortillas. I ask the waitperson to ask the chef to substitute a house salad for the guacamole and rice.

Cactus Special – Grilled chicken or beef on top of rice and smothered in our famous cheese sauce. I ask the waitperson to ask the chef to prepare this dish without the rice.

Polo Monterey – Grilled chicken smothered in onions and peppers with lettuce, sour cream and pico de gallo topped with chili con queso.

Taco Grande – Two large tacos, your choice of beef or chicken topped with lettuce, shredded cheese and tomato. Served with rice and beans. I ask the waitperson to ask the chef to substitute a house salad for the rice and beans.

Sides:

House Salad

Pico de Gallo

Sour Cream

Shredded Cheese

Desserts:

Flan – Caramelized custard with whipped cream.

Fried Ice Cream

Fried Cheesecake Burrito

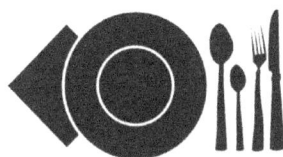

Fast Food Restaurants

Lunch/Dinner

Corner Bakery Café
International Chain Restaurant

Signature Hand Tossed Salads:

Chopped Salad – All-natural chicken, bacon, avocado, blue cheese, tomatoes and green onions with iceberg and romaine lettuce and sweet and spicy vinaigrette. I ask the counterperson to ask the chef to substitute extra tomatoes and green onions for the bacon and avocado.

Santa Fe Ranch – All-natural chicken, roasted corn and tomato salsa and cheddar cheese tossed with iceberg and romaine lettuce, ranch dressing and tortilla strips. I ask the counterperson to ask the chef to leave off the tortilla strips.

Spinach Sweet Crisp – Spinach, strawberries, grapes, cranberries, green onions and creamy goat cheese with raisin pecan sweet crisps and homemade pomegranate vinaigrette.

Asian Wonton – All-natural chicken, edamame, tomatoes, cucumbers, peppers, green onions, cilantro and crispy wontons with mixed greens, cabbage, and ginger soy dressing. I ask the counterperson to ask the chef to substitute extra tomatoes and peppers for the cucumbers and crispy wontons.

Harvest Salad – Green apples, toasted walnuts, blue cheese and currants, tossed with mixed greens, balsamic vinaigrette and harvest crisps. All-natural chicken is available for an additional charge. I ask the waitperson to ask the chef to leave off the harvest crisps.

Homemade Specialty Salads:

The Trio – Create your own handcrafted favorite. Your choice of three freshly made Specialty Salads with field greens. For an additional charge you can add a cup of homemade soup, two specialty salads or field greens.

New! Toasted Sesame Kale – Fresh kale, shredded carrots and toasted sesame seeds with ginger soy dressing.

D.C. Chicken Salad – All-natural chicken, green apples, currants, red onions, celery, mayo and toasted almonds.

Asian Edamame Salad – Edamame, tomatoes, cucumbers, carrots, green onions, peppers, basil and cilantro in ginger soy dressing. I ask the counterperson to ask the chef to substitute extra peppers for the cucumbers.

Mozzarella Tomato Arugula – Marinated tomatoes, fresh mozzarella, arugula and basil with lemon garlic dressing.

Seasonal Fruit Medley

Mixed Greens Salad

Soup & Chili:

Cups and bowls served with freshly baked focaccia roll.

Homemade Soups – Our hot and hearty soups are a perfect addition to any meal.

Big Al's Chili – Our secret recipe topped with sharp cheddar cheese.

Corner Combos:

Sandwich or Panini Combo – Half a sandwich or panini with mixed greens or a cup of soup. For an additional charge substitute Big Al's Chili for a cup of soup.

Signature Salad Combo – Your choice of any Café Size Signature hand-tossed salad with a cup of soup. For an additional charge, substitute Big Al's Chili for a cup of soup.

Signature Sandwiches:

Sandwiches are served with a pickle and bakery chips or baby carrots. For an additional charge you can substitute a mixed green salad for the bakery chips. On all sandwiches I order the baby carrots.

Chicken Pesto – On ciabatta ficelle. All-natural chicken, arugula and tomatoes with our sweet and spicy vinaigrette and pesto mayo.

Uptown Turkey – On harvest toast. Smoked turkey, Applewood smoked bacon, avocado, lettuce, tomatoes and mayo. I ask the counterperson to ask the chef to substitute extra lettuce and tomato for the bacon and avocado.

D.C. Chicken Salad – On steakhouse rye. All-natural chicken, apples, currants, onions, celery, mayo and almonds with lettuce and tomato.

Turkey Pretzel – On pretzel bread. Shaved red onions, tomatoes, caraway Havarti cheese and stoneground mustard-mayo.

Tomato Mozzarella – On ciabatta ficelle. Roasted red peppers, arugula and basil with balsamic vinaigrette.

Mom's Sandwiches:

With leaf lettuce, tomatoes and country Dijon mustard or mayo.

Smoked Turkey on Harvest

Grilled Chicken on Harvest

Hot Toasted Sandwiches:

Served on a toasted French roll with a pickle and bakery chips or baby carrots. I order the baby carrots.

Steak & Cheese – Roast beef and provolone cheese with grilled mushrooms, peppers and onions topped with cheddar sauce and our signature dipping sauce.

Turkey Pastrami – Turkey pastrami, Swiss cheese, creamy coleslaw and Dijon mustard.

Bakery Fresh Sweets:

Cinnamon Crème Cake – Our signature rich, golden cake swirled with ribbons of cinnamon, topped with crumbly cinnamon streusel and powdered sugar.

Bundt Cakes – Available in medium and baby bundt sizes. Available in chocolate and gingerbread pumpkin.

Rugalach – Available in cinnamon pecan and apple walnut.

Dickey's Barbecue Pit
Chain Restaurant

Pit Smoked Meats:

Our meats are seasoned and slow cooked in hickory wood burning pits on-site daily at each of our restaurants.

Beef Brisket – Hickory "smoked to perfection" brisket.

Turkey Breast – Tender and juicy turkey.

Chicken – Savory, Italian marinated chicken breasts.

Home Style Sides:

Our sides have been perfected over the years. We've got the classic barbecue sides.

Creamy Coleslaw

Caesar Salad – I ask the counterperson to ask the chef to substitute another salad dressing for the Caesar dressing and to leave off the croutons.

Sandwiches:

Indulge in one of our 3 sandwich options. Wanna upgrade? Make it a plate and add 2 sides to any sandwich for a special price.

The Westerner – Not to be outdone, this is our largest sandwich with your choice of 2 slow-cooked meats and 2 slices of delicious cheddar cheese.

Big Barbecue – For those looking to satisfy a serious barbecue craving – this is a great option. I ask the counterperson to ask the chef to substitute mustard for the barbecue sauce.

Lil' Hoagie – Little sandwich, big flavor. Have you had your hoagie today?

Meat Plate:

All of our meat plates are served with pickles, onions, barbecue sauce and your choice of 2 home style sides. I ask the counterperson to ask the chef to substitute mustard for the barbecue sauce.

3-Meat Plate – Can't decide? This is the perfect plate to have everything you're craving!

2-Meat Plate – For those looking to satisfy a serious barbecue craving – this is a taste option.

1-Meat Plate – A hearty serving of your favorite meat.

Quarter Plate – For those with a smaller appetite, this is a great way to get your barbecue fix without having to waste a single bite!

Bakers & Salads:

What could be better than taking one of our fresh salads or bakers and topping them off with slow-cooked barbecue? We had a hard time thinking of something too. Try our signature Smokehouse Salad or add any meat to our Giant Baker.

Giant Baker + Meat – Bacon, shredded cheddar, sour cream, margarine & green onions. For a little extra – top it off with any meat. I ask the counter person to ask the chef to leave off the bacon and margarine.

Garden Salad – Romaine lettuce, shredded cheddar cheese, croutons & ranch dressing. I ask the counterperson to ask the chef to substitute extra lettuce for the croutons.

Smokehouse Salad – Chopped beef brisket, romaine lettuce, shredded cheddar, fried onion tanglers & ranch dressing. I ask the counterperson to ask the chef to substitute raw onion for the fried onions.

Chicken Caesar Salad – Sliced chicken, romaine lettuce, shredded parmesan, croutons & Caesar dressing. I ask the counterperson to ask the chef to substitute extra lettuce for the croutons and to substitute ranch dressing for the Caesar dressing.

Family Packs:

Have a lot to feed? Take home a family pack today! The perfect option for tailgate parties, get-togethers, special occasions and more.

Drinks & Desserts:

Fill up your Big Yellow Cup with Miss Ollie Dickey's famous iced tea. Satisfy your sweet tooth one of our assorted dessert options – including pecan pie!

Firehouse Subs
Chain Restaurant

Salad & Chili:

Chief's Salad ® – A blend of romaine and iceberg lettuce topped with bell pepper, cucumber, red onion, tomato, provolone, sliced egg and your choice of meat. I ask the counterperson to ask the chef to substitute extra tomato for the cucumber.

Firehouse Chili – Award-winning.

Hot Specialty Subs:

Firehouse Meatball® – Italian meatballs, melted provolone, zesty marinara, and Italian seasonings.

New York Steamer Sub® – Corned beef brisket, pastrami, melted provolone, mustard, mayo, and Italian dressing.

Firehouse Steak & Cheese® – Sautéed sirloin steak, melted provolone, onions, bell peppers, mayo and mustard.

Engineer Sub® – Smoked turkey breast, melted Swiss, sautéed mushrooms, served Fully Involved.

Smokehouse Beef & Cheddar Brisket® – USDA choice beef brisket smoked for 16+ hours, melted cheddar and special sauces.

Fully Involved®:

Loaded Complete – With mayo, deli mustard, lettuce, tomato, onion and a Kosher dill pickle on the side.

Additional Hot Subs:

All subs served hot with provolone on a toasted sub roll, served Fully Involved®.

Smoked Turkey Breast

Pastrami

Corned Beef Brisket

Premium Roast Beef

Sliced Chicken Breast

Veggie

Cold Subs:

White Chicken Salad

Medium Sub Add-Ons:

Extra Cheese

Mushrooms

Kids' Combos:

Hot Turkey & Provolone

Hot Meatball

KFC
International Chain Restaurant

Grilled Chicken

Grilled Chicken Sandwich

Coleslaw

Green Beans

Milk

Ice Tea – Without the ice. Low calorie sweetener.

La Salsa
Fresh Mexican Grill
Chain Restaurant

La Salsa's approach to the best Mexican food possible is simple. We take time honored, authentic Mexican dishes and update them using the freshest ingredients and preparation to bring the bold tastes and flavors of Mexico to life in a variety of unique ways. We're constantly exploring, trying new tastes and ideas, and updating our menu so that we can share with you our twists on the flavors of Mexico's varied regions.

Experience the sights, sounds, smells and tastes of the taqueria-fresh Mexican food menu at La Salsa Fresh Mexican Grill.

Tacos:

Mexico City Tacos – Inspired by authentic Mexican street tacos, Mexico City Tacos are soft taco shells stuffed with grilled chicken, carne asada or carnitas and topped with fresh cilantro and onion. Choose any combination of three you'd like. Includes rice, beans and chips. I eat either the beans or rice on a reward day.

Tacos La Salsa® -Clearly a favorite of ours… Two giant tacos stuffed with grilled chicken and topped with jack and cheddar cheeses and fresh lettuce and tomatoes.

Burritos:

Overstuffed Grilled Burrito – A heaping double-portion of chicken, habanero jack cheese, fresh salsa and guacamole all packed into a flour tortilla and grilled up to a two handed perfection. I ask the counterperson to ask the chef to substitute extra cheese for the guacamole.

NO Rice NO Beans™ Burrito – But lots of meat and veggies-grilled chicken, fajita veggies, zucchini, broccoli, carrots, corn and salsa combined with habanero jack cheese and poblano crema and then wrapped up tight in a flour tortilla. I ask the counterperson to ask the chef to substitute extra broccoli for the corn.

Salads:

Chile-Lime Salad – Fresh, crispy romaine lettuce loaded with grilled chicken, cotija cheese, fresh tomatoes and avocado and topped with chile-lime dressing and tortilla strips. I ask the counterperson to ask the chef to substitute extra tomatoes for the avocado and to leave off the tortilla strips.

Platters:

Two Tacos La Salsa® – Our Favorite, Tacos La Salsa- Two giant tacos stuffed with grilled chicken and topped with jack and cheddar cheeses and fresh lettuce and tomatoes.

Enchilada – A pair of fresh corn tortillas wrapped around a blend of jack and cheddar cheeses smothered in rioja sauce and topped with melted cheeses and crema Mexicana.

Three Pepper Fajita -Your choice of grilled chicken or juicy strips of sirloin steak served with fire-roasted fajita veggies and toppings of fresh guacamole, cheese and sour cream, and piping hot corn or flour tortillas to wrap it all up in. I ask the counterperson to ask the chef to substitute extra fire-roasted veggies for the guacamole.

McDonalds
International Chain Restaurant

Burgers & Sandwiches:

Delicious, freshly made, and oh-so-satisfying. From the Big Mac to our Premium Grilled Chicken Club to our Classic Cheeseburger, McDonalds sandwiches make the meal. Not all establishments will do it, but when they will let me I ask the counterperson to make the substitutions listed below.

Hamburger

Cheeseburger – I ask the waitperson to ask the grill chef to substitute cheddar for American cheese.

Grilled Onion Cheddar Burger

Premium Grilled Chicken Classic Sandwich

Premium McWrap Southwest (Grilled)

Premium McWrap Chicken & Ranch (Grilled)

Premium McWrap Sweet Chili Chicken (Grilled)

Salads:

Can salads be classy? We say yes. Add a little panache to your day with select mixed greens, elegant toppings and choices galore.

Premium Bacon Ranch Salad – I ask the counterperson to ask the grill cook to substitute extra lettuce for the bacon.

Premium Bacon Ranch Salad with Grilled Chicken – I ask the counterperson to ask the grill cook to substitute extra lettuce for the bacon.

Premium Southwest Salad

Premium Southwest Salad with Grilled Chicken

Side Salad

Noodles & Company
Chain Restaurant

Sandwiches:

The Med – Grilled chicken, mushrooms, spinach, red bell pepper, cucumber, red onion, our zesty Med dressing, cilantro and feta on flat bread. I ask the counterperson to ask the chef to substitute extra spinach for the cucumber.

Wisconsin Cheesesteak – Marinated steak, our mac and cheese sauce, cheddar and Jack cheese, red onion, red bell pepper and mushrooms on ciabatta.

Salads:

Spinach & Fresh Fruit Salad – Seasonal fruit, crumbled bacon, pecans, house-made croutons, red onion and blue cheese atop spinach with a balsamic fig drizzle. I ask the counterperson to ask the chef to substitute extra spinach for the bacon and croutons.

Grilled Chicken Caesar – Grilled chicken, romaine, croutons, traditional dressing and parmesan. I ask the counterperson to ask the chef to substitute extra romaine for the croutons and to substitute balsamic vinaigrette for the Caesar dressing.

Chinese Chicken Chop Salad – Grilled chicken, sesame-soy tossed mixed greens, Asian sprouts, cabbage, red bell pepper, cucumber, carrots, crispy wontons and black sesame seeds. I ask the counterperson to ask the chef to substitute extra mixed greens for the cucumber and the wontons.

The Med Salad with Chicken – Grilled chicken, romaine, mixed greens, tomato, cucumber, red onion, olives, cavatappi pasta, spicy yogurt dressing and feta. I ask the counterperson to ask the chef to substitute extra romaine for the cucumber.

Featured Dish:

Alfredo MontAmore® – Spaghetti noodles, four-cheese blend, mushrooms, spinach, tomato, and parmesan chicken. Topped with MontAmore cheese, parsley and cracked pepper.

Noodles & Pasta:

Can add grilled or parmesan chicken for an additional charge.

Penne Rosa- Spicy tomato cream sauce, penne pasta, mushrooms, tomato, spinach, wine and parmesan or feta.

Japanese Pan Noodles – Caramelized udon noodles in a sweet soy sauce, broccoli, carrots, shitake mushrooms Asian sprouts, black sesame seeds and cilantro.

Pesto Cavatappi – Curly pasta, basil pesto, garlic, mushrooms, tomato, wine, cream, parmesan and Italian parsley.

Spaghetti & Meatballs – five meatballs on spaghetti, crushed tomato marinara and parmesan.

Pasta Fresca – Penne with balsamic, olive oil, white wine and roasted garlic, red onion, tomato, spinach and parmesan or feta.

Steak Stroganoff – Marinated steak, mushroom sherry cream sauce, fresh herbs, cracked pepper, sautéed mushrooms, egg noodles and parmesan.

Whole Grain Tuscan Linguine – Whole grain linguine, broccoli, red bell pepper, onion, mushrooms, garlic, white wine, cream and parmesan.

Soups:

Tomato Basil Bisque – Rich zesty tomato soup with cream, sherry, fresh basil, garlic, and Italian parsley.

Pita Taza Mediterranean Grill
Albuquerque, NM

All fresh ingredients – kosher lamb and beef.

Appetizers:

I do not eat the pita bread.

Ba'ba Ghannoug – Baked eggplant, mashed and blended with tahini, yogurt & parsley, topped with olive oil & spices. Served as a cold dip with pita bread.

Jerusalem Salad – Freshly diced tomatoes, cucumbers & parsley. Dressed with our own special tahini sauce. I ask the counterperson to ask the chef to substitute diced green pepper for the cucumbers.

Greek Feta Cheese Salad – Freshly diced tomatoes, onions, parsley, green pepper & cracked wheat gently tossed with olive oil & lemon juice. I ask the counterperson to ask the chef to leave out the cracked wheat.

Fatoush Salad – Lettuce, tomatoes, cucumbers, onions & green peppers tossed in our house vinaigrette & topped with our homemade pita croutons. I ask the counterperson to ask the chef to substitute extra tomatoes for the cucumbers and pita croutons.

Sandwiches:

All are served with French fries. On all sandwiches I ask the counterperson to ask the chef to substitute a Fatoush Salad for the French Fries.

Lamb Shish Kabob – Grilled pieces of marinated kosher lamb, served in a pita pocket with lettuce and tomato.

Kifta Kabob Sandwich – Grilled & seasoned ground cuts of tender beef, onion, parsley, served in a pita pocket with lettuce & tomato.

Beef Shawarma Sandwich – Thin slices of lightly seasoned beef cooked on a slowly revolving rotisserie, served in a pita pocket with lettuce, tomato & tahini sauce.

Chicken Kabob Sandwich – Marinated Mediterranean style chicken breast, grilled & served in a pita pocket with lettuce & tomato.

Falafel Sandwich – Seasoned ground chick peas & vegetables, formed into patties & deep fried to a flavorful crispness, served in a pita pocket with lettuce, tomato & tahini sauce. I eat falafel sandwiches on reward days.

Kosher Gyros Sandwich – A generous portion of our famous gyros served on a pita bread with our delicious sauce, onions & tomato.

Cheeseburger – American cheese, lettuce, pickles, tomato & sauce. I ask the counterperson to ask the chef to substitute feta cheese for the American cheese.

Entrees:

Served with rice pilaf, salad & pita bread. On all entrees I ask the counterperson to ask the chef to substitute an extra salad for the rice.

Lamb Shish Kabob – Grilled pieces of tender kosher lamb.

Kifta Kabob – Grilled seasoned ground cuts of tender beef, minced onion & parsley.

Beef Shawarma – Thin slices of slightly seasoned beef cooked on a slowly revolving rotisserie.

Chicken Kabob – Marinated & grilled Mediterranean style chicken breast.

Combination Feast – Combination of shish kabob, Kifta kabob & Shawarma. (Add a chicken kabob for an additional charge.)

Hummus & Shawarma – A blend of ground chick peas &

tahini, topped with beef or chicken Shawarma.

Vegetarian Falafel Plate – Seasoned ground chick peas & vegetables, formed into patties then deep fried to a flavorful crispness. Served with tahini sauce, hot sauce, lettuce & tomato. I eat this dish on a reward night.

Kosher Gyros Plate – Thin slices of slightly seasoned beef cooked on a slowly revolving rotisserie.

Desserts:

Baklava

Kinafa

Dessert of the day

Steak n' Shake
International Chain Restaurant

Sandwiches:

Turkey Club Sandwich – Oven-roasted turkey breast, Applewood smoked bacon, crisp lettuce, vine-ripened tomato and mayo on two slices of Texas toast. Served with fries. I ask the waitperson to ask the chef to substitute extra lettuce and tomatoes for the bacon and to substitute coleslaw for the fries. I also ask the waitperson to ask the chef to serve the sandwich open face.

Jalapeno Crunch Chicken Sandwich – Marinated grilled chicken breast topped with pepper Jack cheese, chipotle mayo, fresh salsa and jalapenos, all topped with Frenches French fried onions. Served with fries. I ask the waitperson to ask the chef to substitute grilled onions for the French fried onions and to substitute a garden salad for the fries.

Grilled Chicken Sandwich- A marinated grilled chicken breast topped with crisp lettuce, vine-ripened tomato and mayo. Served with fries. I ask the waitperson to ask the chef to substitute coleslaw for the fries.

Salads:

Dressings: Ranch, honey mustard, gourmet bleu cheese, and zesty Italian.

Apple Harvest Grilled Chicken Salad – Crispy lettuce blend topped with plenty of fresh ingredients – fresh apple, Roma tomato, avocado, chopped almonds and Ocean Spray® dried cranberries plus a diced, warm, grilled chicken breast. Served with reduced fat berry balsamic vinaigrette. I ask the waitperson to ask the chef to substitute bleu cheese dressing for the balsamic vinaigrette and to substitute extra apple for the avocado.

Taco Salad – Enjoy the flavors of the Southwest. We begin with our Steakburger ™ beef, expertly seasoned and served over crispy lettuce with diced tomato, shredded cheese, crispy tortilla strips, and ranch dressing. I ask the waitperson to ask the chef to leave off the tortilla strips.

Grilled Chicken Salad – Marinated, grilled chicken breast served warm over our crispy lettuce blend, along with freshly grated carrots, red cabbage, diced tomatoes, cheddar n' Jack cheese, croutons, and your choice of dressing. I ask the waitperson to ask the chef to leave off the croutons.

Sides:

Vegetable Soup

Genuine Chili

Creamy Coleslaw

Garden Salad

Genuine Chili:

Made with 100% beef, plump beans and a blend of spices, slow-simmered according to our founder's wife's recipe.

Genuine Chili – Chili beef, chili beans and our blend of special seasonings.

Chili Deluxe – Our Genuine Chili with diced, fresh onions and shredded cheddar n' Jack cheese.

Classic Melts:

Buttery crisp grilled bread on the outside, and a warm cheesy inside. A Steak 'n Shake signature. Served with fries. On all melts I ask the waitperson to ask the chef to substitute a garden salad for the fries.

Frisco Melt – Two Steakburgers™ with American and Swiss cheeses on buttery grilled sourdough with our sweet 'n tangy

Frisco sauce. I ask the waitperson to ask the chef to substitute extra Swiss for the American cheese.

Patty Melt – Two Steakburgers™ with American cheese and caramelized onions melted together on toasty, grilled rye. I ask the waitperson to ask the chef to substitute Swiss for American cheese.

Pepper Jack Melt – Two Steakburgers™ with melted pepper Jack cheese, lettuce, vine-ripened tomato, grilled onions, jalapenos, and mayo on grilled sourdough – just the right amount of spicy.

Chicken Melt – Grilled chicken, melted Swiss cheese, vine-ripened tomato, Applewood smoked bacon and our sweet 'n tangy Frisco sauce on grilled sourdough. I ask the waitperson to ask the chef to substitute extra tomato for the bacon.

Veggie Melt – Melted pepper Jack cheese, leaf lettuce, vine-ripened tomatoes, homemade guacamole, red onions and Portobello mushrooms all served on sourdough. I ask the waitperson to ask the chef to substitute extra lettuce and tomato for the guacamole.

Steakburger Shooters®

Mini Steakburgers made with 100% beef. Combine your favorite shooters!

Add a Side:

Creamy Coleslaw

Garden Salad

Cup of Soup or Chili

The Original Steakburger™:

Made with 100% beef, which includes steak, quick seared on our fiery-hot grill to seal in the flavor and create our unique crispy edges. Served on a toasted bun with fries. I ask the waitperson to substitute a garden salad for the fries on all Steakburgers ™.

The Original Double, N Cheese – Our most popular Steakburger! Two hot-off-the-grill Steakburgers™ with American Cheese, fresh lettuce, pickles, vine-ripened tomato, onion, and ketchup. I ask the waitperson to ask the chef to substitute Swiss for the American cheese and to substitute mustard for the ketchup.

Bacon 'n Cheese Double Steakburger™ – I ask the waitperson to ask the chef to substitute lettuce and tomato for the bacon.

Single Steakburger™

Triple Steakburger™

Grilled Portobello 'n Swiss Steakburger™ – A double Steakburger™ with fresh Portobello mushrooms, seasoned on our fiery-hot grill and topped with melted Swiss cheese, caramelized onions, garlic and mayo.

Cheesy Cheddar Steakburger™ – A double Steakburger™ smothered with loads of melted Wisconsin cheddar – a cheese lover's delight. Served with lettuce and vine-ripened tomato.

Hand-Dipped Milkshakes:

Classics – Hand-dipped, real milk and classic flavors. Chocolate. Strawberry. Vanilla.

Whataburger
Chain Restaurant

Burgers:

Meals served with French Fries or apple slices and a 32 oz. drink. I order the apple slices and iced tea.

Whataburger – Includes mustard, lettuce, tomatoes, pickles on a toasted 5" bun.

Double Meat Whataburger

Chicken:

Meals served with French Fries or apple slices and a 32 oz. drink. I order the apple slices and iced tea.

Whatachick 'n' Sandwich – Includes lettuce, tomatoes and mayo on a whole grain bun.

Grilled Chicken Sandwich – Includes lettuce, tomatoes and mayo on a whole grain bun.

Chicken Fajita Taco – Grilled chicken breast with grilled onions, poblano and red bell peppers.

Grilled Chicken Melt – Comes with grilled onions, poblano and red bell peppers and Monterey Jack cheese.

All-Time Favorites:

All-Time Favorites meals served with French Fries or apple slices and a 32 oz. drink. I order the apple slices and iced tea.

Whataburger Patty Melt – Two 100% beef patties, grilled onions and two slices of Monterey Jack cheese topped with our famous Creamy Pepper Sauce.

Monterey Melt – Two 100 beef patties, melted slices of American and Monterey Jack cheese, jalapeno ranch and a blend of grilled onions, poblano peppers and red bell peppers. I ask the counterperson to ask the grill cook to substitute extra Monterey Jack cheese for the American cheese.

Add-Ons:

Green Chiles

Cheese

Grilled Peppers & Onions

Dipping Sauces:

Creamy Pepper

Honey Mustard

Ranch

Sides:

Apple Slices – Comes in a 2 oz. package.

Salads:

Apple & Cranberry Chicken Salad – Romaine lettuce, dried cranberries, crispy apples and shredded cheddar cheese topped with grilled chicken.

Garden Salad – Romaine lettuce, grape tomatoes, shredded carrots and cheddar cheese. Add grilled chicken.

Whole Hog Café
Santa Fe & Albuquerque, NM
North Little Rock & Bryant, AR

Sandwiches:

All sandwiches are garnished with coleslaw. All meats are dry rubbed with spices and smoked with pecan wood.

Beef Brisket

Pulled Chicken

Plates:

Includes meat, 2 side orders and a dinner roll.

Beef Brisket

Pulled Chicken

Half Chicken

Salads:

Salad – Iceberg/Romaine lettuce.

Barbecue Salad – Pulled chicken or beef.

Choice of Dressing – Ranch, Italian, Blue Cheese, Honey Mustard, Fat Free Raspberry Vinaigrette.

Side Orders:

Coleslaw

Salad

Desserts:

Brownies

Chocolate Sheet Cake

Chocolate Mousse Pie

Bulk Meats to Go:

Beef Brisket

Pulled Chicken

Half Chicken

Sides – See above listing.

Wild Smoke
Creve Coeur, MO

Soup and Salads:

For an additional charge you can add pulled chicken or brisket to any salad.

Smoked Chicken Tortilla Soup

BBQ Chicken Salad – With ranch dressing.

Waco Wedge – With blue cheese dressing

Side Salad – With roasted garlic lemon vinaigrette on the side.

Platters:

Choice of 2 sides.

Pulled Chicken

Smoked Turkey

Beef Brisket

Prime Rib

Sideshow:

Slaw

Grilled Green Beans

Two Meat Combo:

Choose any two meats: pulled chicken, brisket, or turkey.

Backyard Favorites:

Smoked Half Chicken – Seasoned and wood grilled.

Dessert:

Soft Brownie

Kentucky Bourbon Pecan Pie

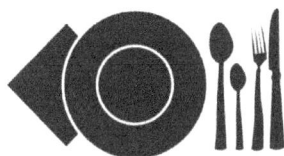

HOTEL DINING

BREAKFAST

Sheraton
Hotel Chain

Chef's Omelet – Cured ham, sliced mushrooms, sweet onions and aged cheddar and Swiss cheese, served with hash browns. I ask the waitperson to ask the chef to substitute extra mushrooms for the cured ham.

Egg White, Tomato & Spinach Omelet – Folded with white cheddar cheese and cured over tomatoes.

Open Faced Breakfast Sandwich – Scrambled eggs and Canadian bacon on an English muffin with onions, tomato and white cheddar cheese served with hash brown potatoes. I ask the waitperson to ask the chef to substitute extra tomato and onion for the bacon.

Bounty of Fruits & Berries – Seasonal selection of market's best served with low-fat yogurt. I ask the waitperson to ask the chef to substitute cheddar cheese for the yogurt.

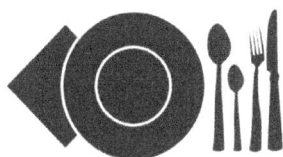

HOTEL DINING

LUNCH/DINNER

The French Pastry Shop
La Fonda
Albuquerque, NM

Savory Crepes:

Ratatouille – Zucchini, eggplant, tomatoes, onions and green peppers.

Chicken Mushroom – With béchamel sauce.

Chicken Mushroom – With béchamel sauce & spinach.

Spinach & Cheese

Hot Sandwiches:

Croque Monsieur – Ham, cheese, béchamel sauce. I ask the waitperson to ask the chef to substitute chicken for the ham.

Sandwiches on Baguette:

Half & Full size available. Swiss cheese is available for an extra charge.

Roast Beef

Turkey

Quick French Meals:

Spinach Quiche

Dinner Salad – I ask the waitperson to ask the chef to prepare my salad without any cucumbers or croutons.

French Onion Soup – I ask the waitperson to ask the chef to prepare my soup without any bread or croutons.

Soup Special

<u>Sweet Crepes:</u>

Nutella, vanilla ice cream, chocolate syrup & whipped cream are available for an additional charge.

<u>Strawberry</u>

<u>Blueberry</u>

<u>Raspberry</u>

<u>Peach</u>

<u>Apricot</u>

<u>Cherry</u>

<u>Fruit Combinations</u>

<u>Nutella</u>

La Plazuela Restaurant
La Fonda Hotel
Albuquerque, NM

Appetizers, Soups and Salads:

Quesadilla – Your choice of flour or wheat tortillas filled with grilled squashes, white beans, mushrooms, and Monterey Jack cheese and served with green chile sauce. Chicken breast can be added for an additional charge. I ask the waitperson to ask the chef to substitute additional squash for the white beans.

La Plazuela Tortilla Soup – Roasted tomato-pasilla chile chicken broth with shredded chicken, Mexican cheeses, avocado and lime tortilla strips. I ask the waitperson to ask the chef to substitute extra Mexican cheese for the avocado and to substitute a lime for the tortilla strips.

Venison Texas Chile – Hearty ground venison, red onions and tomato, served with jalapeno cheddar cornbread.

La Fonda Cobb – Chopped and stacked romaine hearts, roasted turkey breast, seasonal tomatoes, avocado, jicama, Applewood smoked bacon and blue cheese tossed with apple cider vinaigrette. I ask the waitperson to ask the chef to substitute extra romaine hearts for the avocado and the bacon.

La Fonda Caesar Salad – Fresh romaine hearts tossed with Cotija Caesar dressing and garnished with seasonal tomatoes, red onion slices and sourdough croutons. Chicken breast can be added for an additional charge. I ask the waitperson to ask the chef to substitute blue cheese dressing for the Caesar dressing and to substitute extra tomatoes for the sourdough croutons.

Spinach Salad – Baby spinach tossed with hot bacon

dressing and red onions, topped with sliced hard boiled eggs and local feta cheese. I ask the waitperson to ask the chef to substitute blue cheese dressing for the hot bacon dressing.

La Plazuela Sandwiches:

Served with a house side salad and a pickle.

Torta de Borrego – Tender local Felix River Ranch lamb shoulder, braised and served on a toasted Telera bread topped with sliced seasonal tomatoes, sliced avocado, caramelized onions, arugula, local feta cheese and lemon-cilantro aioli. I ask the waitperson to ask the chef to substitute extra tomato for the avocado.

Turkey Club Wrap – Roasted turkey breast served in a flour or wheat tortilla, filled with crispy Applewood smoked bacon, pico de gallo, roasted garlic aioli and shredded lettuce. I ask the waitperson to ask the chef to substitute extra turkey for the bacon.

Hatch Green Chile Cheeseburger – Freshly ground all-natural New Mexico beef patty grilled to order topped with roasted Hatch green chile served on a Telera bun with your choice of Swiss or cheddar cheese.

Dinner Menu:

The same as above.

Specialties of the Chef:

Filet Mignon – Char-grilled 6 oz. center-cut petite beef tenderloin, served with chanterelle mushroom demi-glace, roasted garlic buttermilk mashed potatoes and seasonal vegetables. I ask the waitperson to ask the chef to substitute extra seasonal vegetables for the mashed potatoes.

Santa Fe Meatloaf – Ground New Mexico beef filled with

local Hatch green chile, raisins and pinion, baked with spicy ketchup glaze and served with smoked tomato coulis, roasted garlic buttermilk mashed potatoes and seasonal vegetables. I ask the waitperson to ask the chef to substitute extra seasonal vegetables for the mashed potatoes.

Organic Chicken Breast – Pan-roasted chicken breast with mole negro served with creamy sweet potato polenta and fresh seasonal vegetables. I ask the waitperson to ask the chef to substitute extra vegetables for the sweet potato polenta.

Northern New Mexico Specialties:

All, except for tacos, are served with your choice of pico de gallo, sour cream, shredded lettuce and sopaipillas.

Filet y Enchiladas – Char-grilled petite filet mignon served with two Mexican cheese enchiladas topped with your choice of local Hatch red, green or Christmas chile.

Enchiladas del Norte – Two rolled yellow tortillas filled with your choice of shredded beef, chicken or Mexican cheeses topped with your choice of local Hatch red, green or Christmas chile. Add two eggs for an additional charge.

Burrito de La Plazuela – A flour filled tortilla with your choice of shredded beef or chicken topped with your choice of local Hatch red, green or Christmas chile.

Fajitas de Santa Fe – Your choice of marinated and grilled beef skirt steak or chicken breast or a combination with bell peppers, sweet Spanish onions, served with corn or flour tortillas.

Mas Tapas y Vino
Hotel Andaluz
Albuquerque, NM

Mas Tapas:

Spiced Almonds

Olives, Grapes and Garlic

Quinoa Salad – Pomegranate, parsley, grilled avocado, pimento yogurt. I ask the waitperson to ask the chef to substitute extra pomegranate for the grilled avocado.

Grilled Eggplant, melted Manchego, capers, and saffron honey.

Manchengo Cheese with Membrillo

Grilled Artichokes – With Spanish goat cheese, orange zest & mint.

Mezze Platter – Carrot-garbanzo hummus, beet-walnut spread, roasted eggplant puree and sesame-lavash crackers.

Spanish Cheese Plate – Manchengo, goat cheese, cabrales, almonds, figs, and membrillo.

Queso Fresco – Manzanilla olives, dried figs, chile flake, and olive oil.

Hot Gouda – Chorizo, apple baked with crostini. I ask the waitperson to ask the chef to leave off the chorizo.

Roasted Duck Breast – With tart cherry mostarda.

Grilled Lamb Chops – With harissa, cucumber, yogurt and dill. I ask the waitperson to ask the chef to leave off the cucumber.

Grilled NM Flatiron Steak – With smoky sea salt caramel.

Chef's Daily Soup:

Salads:

Can add chicken for an additional charge.

Roasted Beet & Spanish Goat Cheese Salad – Baby greens with pomegranate vinaigrette.

Kale & Baby Spinach Salad – Fried garbanzo beans with rhubarb-bacon vinaigrette. I ask the waitperson to ask the chef to sauté the garbanzo beans and to substitute a vinaigrette that does not have bacon.

Heirloom Tomato & Fresh Mozzarella Salad – Basil-mint vinaigrette with sherry vinegar reduction.

Grilled Flatiron Steak Salad – Grilled asparagus, cabrales blue cheese, and charred tomato vinaigrette.

Quinoa Salad – Parsley, pomegranate seeds, grilled avocado, and pimento yogurt. I ask the waitperson to ask the chef to substitute grilled asparagus for the grilled avocado.

Mediterranean Salad – Baby greens, apricots, figs, local feta, and sherry-honey vinaigrette.

Green Apple Manchengo Salad – Marcona almonds and rosemary-cider vinaigrette.

MAS Chopped Chicken Salad – Cucumbers, tomatoes, peppers, manzanilla olives, and preserved lemon-yogurt dressing. I ask the waitperson to ask the chef to substitute extra tomatoes for the cucumbers.

Sandwiches:

Served with side salad, or fruit. Can have any **1/2** sandwich with a cup of soup. I order either the **1/2** sandwich with a cup of soup or the whole sandwich with a side salad.

Grilled Vegetable Hummus Wrap – Zucchini, squash, onions, peppers, eggplant, carrot-garbanzo hummus, and goat cheese.

Tomato-Mozzarella Sandwich – Basil-mint pesto on house made focaccia.

Turkey Cheddar Green Chile Panini – Avocado with green olive aioli. I ask the waitperson to ask the chef to substitute tomato for the avocado.

Chicken Harissa Wrap – Baby spinach, feta, roasted red peppers, and harissa sauce.

Burgers:

Choice of sides: soup, side salad, or fruit.

Mas Burger – Crispy jamon serrano, cabrales blue cheese and olive aioli. I ask the waitperson to ask the chef to substitute tomato for the crispy jamon serrano.

NM Green Chile Cheeseburger – Cheddar, lettuce, tomato, and onion.

Coca-Spanish Flatbreads:

Mushroom Coca – Sautéed mushrooms, melted Manchego, sage, and truffle oil.

Artichoke Coca – Red peppers, goat cheese, and olives.

Platos:

NM Flatiron Steak – Fingerling potatoes and mojo Colorado.

Menu del dia – Special 3 course lunch. Changes daily.

Dinner:

Same menu as listed above.

Tapas:

Grilled NM flatiron steak with smoky sea salt caramel.

Soups:

Chef's sopa de la noche

Entrees:

Roasted duck breast – Moroccan carrot sauce and green couscous. I ask the waitperson to ask the chef to substitute a side salad for the couscous.

8 oz. Filet Mignon – Cabrales butter, Crimini mushrooms, and jamon wrapped asparagus.

NM Flat Iron Steak – Grilled with rosemary rub, herbed fingerlings, baby carrots and tempranillo syrup.

Grilled Lamb Chops – Garlic mint agridulce and winter squash cazuela.

Canelones – pasta stuffed with chicken, red peppers, roasted shallots, Manchego cream, grilled vegetables and sherry vinegar reduction. I eat canelones on a reward night.

Desserts:

Chocolate al Vapor – Steamed chocolate cake with pomegranate chocolate ganache and whipped cream.

Cream Catalana – Baked Spanish custard with vanilla bean and orange essence.

Sheraton
International Hotel Chain

Starters:

House-made Red Pepper Hummus – With a selection of cured olives, roasted peppers and flatbread. I do not eat the flatbread.

Chicken Quesadilla – Amish chicken, poblano peppers, onions, white beans, pepper jack cheese, herb and garlic tortilla. I ask the waitperson to ask the chef to substitute extra onions for the white beans.

Salads:

Chopped Salad with Herb Vinaigrette – Romaine and baby greens, tomato, blue cheese, cucumber, Kalamata olives, onions, sweet peppers, bacon, white beans, croutons, and herb vinaigrette. I ask the waitperson to ask the chef to substitute extra romaine and tomato for the cucumber, bacon, white beans, and croutons.

Caesar Salad – With garlic croutons. I ask the waitperson to ask the chef to leave off the croutons and to substitute blue cheese dressing for the Caesar dressing.

Cobb Salad – Field greens, bacon, avocado, boiled egg, tomato, chicken, and blue cheese. I ask the waitperson to ask the chef to substitute extra field greens and tomato for the bacon and avocado.

Main Courses:

Grilled New York Steak – With crispy onion straws. I ask the waitperson to ask the chef to substitute grilled onions for the onion straws.

Grilled Beef Tenderloin – With golden potatoes, roasted vegetables and cabernet jus. I ask the waitperson to ask the chef to substitute extra roasted vegetables for the potatoes.

Rain Crow Ranch Marinated Grilled Grass-fed-Hanger Steak-
With herb butter.

Cheese Tortellini with Grilled Chicken – Summer vegetables,
chicken broth and sun-dried tomato pesto.

Roasted Chicken Breast – Stuffed with Ozark Forest
Mushrooms, spinach, and goat cheese with creamy white
polenta.

Harvest Vegetable Stack – Vegetable patties with portabella
mushroom, asparagus, red pepper, broccoli, carrot and spinach
with basil pesto.

Grilled Herb Marinated Chicken Breast – Roasted baby
potatoes, harvest vegetables and savory citrus jus. I ask the
waitperson to ask the chef to substitute extra harvest
vegetables for the potatoes.

Sandwiches:

All sandwiches are served with fruit and berry compote.

Herb-roasted Turkey Sandwich – Breast meat, multi-grain
bread, bacon, and house aioli. I ask the waitperson to ask the
chef to substitute lettuce for the bacon.

Chicken Caesar Wrap – Tomato wrap, grilled chicken breast,
romaine lettuce, Parmesan cheese, and Caesar dressing. I ask
the waitperson to ask the chef to substitute blue cheese
dressing for the Caesar dressing.

Grilled Chicken Breast & Provolone Melt – Vine-ripened
tomato, lettuce and red onion on a crusty whole-grain bun.

Little Extras:

Grilled Vegetables

Fruit and Berry Compote

Desserts:

Warm Chocolate Cake – With cinnamon ice cream.

Selection of Ice Creams & Sorbets

Vanilla Crème Brulee – With cinnamon cookies.

Bounty of Berries from the Market

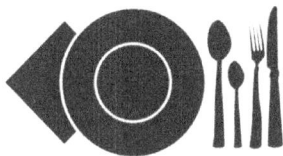

ROOM SERVICE FOOD

ORDER INN® HOSPITALITY SERVICES
Room Service Menu – Serving lunch and dinner
Chain Service Provider

Appetizers & Sides:

Chicken Strips – Available in regular, buffalo style or BBQ.

Garden Fresh Salads:

Dressings: Raspberry Vinaigrette, Ranch, Bleu Cheese, Italian & Greek.

Side Salad – Mixed Greens, cucumber & tomato. I request that extra tomato be substituted for the cucumber and the croutons be left off.

Side Salad w/ Chicken or Gyro Meat

Garden Salad – Mixed greens, cucumber, tomato & green pepper. I request that extra tomato be substituted for the cucumber and the croutons be left off.

Garden Salad w/ Chicken or Gyro Meat

House Special Salad – Mixed greens, cucumber, tomato, green pepper, black olives, pepperoni, mozzarella cheese, pepperoncini peppers, Romano cheese & croutons. I request that extra tomatoes be substituted for the cucumbers, chicken be substituted for the pepperoni, and the croutons be left off.

House Special Salad w/ Chicken or Gyro Meat – I order this salad with chicken and request that Gyro meat be substituted for the pepperoni.

Greek Salad – Mixed greens, cucumber, tomato, green pepper, red onion, Greek olives, banana peppers & feta cheese. I ask the order taker to ask the chef to substitute extra green pepper for the cucumber

Greek Salad w/ Chicken or Gyro Meat

Sandwiches:

All sandwiches are served a la carte on a 6" French roll (except the chicken sandwich).

Gyro – A lamb & beef combination served on pita bread with onion, tomato & gyro sauce.

Italian Beef – Sliced thin & piled high.

Grilled Chicken Breast – Topped with melted mozzarella cheese, lettuce, tomato & mayo.

Pasta:

Served w/ breadsticks & grated cheese. Meat sauce available upon request. (Meat sauce contains ground beef. I do not eat the breadsticks.

Add meat sauce to your pasta for an extra charge.

Spaghetti or Mostaccioli w/ Marinara Sauce

Mostaccioli w/ Chicken – Served with marinara sauce and 1 chicken breast.

Baked Mostaccioli w/ Chicken – Served with marinara sauce and 1 chicken breast.

Baked Lasagna – Homemade from the family recipe. Four layers of mozzarella, ricotta & Romano cheeses, smothered in a delicious marinara sauce.

Baked Lasagna – With 1 chicken breast.

Pizza:

Thin Crust – Choose from the following toppings: artichoke hearts, Italian beef, hamburger, mushrooms, green peppers, feta cheese, gyro meat, ricotta cheese, spinach, onion, Roma tomatoes, fresh garlic, chicken, roasted red peppers and green olives.

Famous Gourmet Pizzas:

Our light, flaky thin crust is always crisp & golden brown.

Spinach Trio Pizza – Spinach, Roma tomatoes, & feta cheese.

Pizza Blanco – Olive oil, fresh garlic, spinach & tomatoes (no red sauce).

The Veggie Pizza – Mushroom, onion, green pepper & sliced tomato.

Chicken Alfredo Pizza – Homemade Alfredo sauce, grilled chicken & sautéed onions. For a different flavor I ask to have marinara sauce substituted for the Alfredo sauce.

Desserts:

Brownies – A 3 oz. brownie w/rich chocolate chunks.

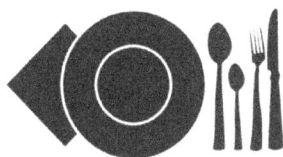

Sports Taverns

Fox & Hound
Chain Restaurant

Pre-Game:

Pile-High Nachos – White corn tortilla chips, cheddar and Monterey jack cheese, queso, lime sour cream, pico de gallo, jalapeños, served with chicken or chili. I ask the waitperson to ask the chef to leave off the jalapenos.

Spinach Artichoke Dip – Spinach, artichoke hearts, three cheeses, roasted garlic, served with chips and salsa

Hummus – Served with toasted pita bread, celery, red peppers, cucumbers & choose your style: Greek: tomatoes, feta cheese, parsley or Buffalo: classic buffalo sauce, bleu cheese crumbles and green onions. I ask the waitperson to ask the chef to substitute extra tomatoes for the cucumbers.

Flatbreads:

Classic Cheese – Mozzarella cheese & oregano.

BBQ Chicken – Chicken, honey BBQ sauce, red onions, pepper Jack cheese, and fresh cilantro.

Lunch:

Chicken Street Tacos – Shredded seasoned chicken, cheddar and Monterey Jack cheeses, pico de gallo, grilled white corn tortilla, served with chips & salsa. For an additional charge can substitute steak. I ask the waitperson to ask the chef to substitute a vegetable for the chips and salsa.

Black Forest – Grilled turkey, Bavarian pretzel roll, Applewood smoked bacon, Monterey Jack cheese, lettuce, tomatoes, honey mustard, served with fries. I ask the waitperson to ask the chef to substitute extra tomato for the bacon and to substitute a vegetable for the fries.

Classic Cheeseburger – Angus burger, lettuce, tomato, pickles, onions, choice of Swiss, cheddar, pepper Jack, American, provolone, or Monterey Jack cheese, served with fries. I order any cheese except American and ask the waitperson to ask the chef to substitute a vegetable for the fries.

Half Flatbread + Salad – choice of classic flatbread and choice of side garden or side Caesar salad. I order the garden salad.

Main Event:

Tavern Glazed Chicken – Two grilled chicken breasts, sesame ginger glaze, green onions, sesame seeds, served with broccoli and rice. I ask the waitperson to ask the chef to substitute a vegetable for the rice.

14oz Ribeye – Grilled USDA center cut choice steak, served with fries and broccoli. I ask the waitperson to ask the chef to substitute a vegetable for the fries.

The Greens:

Hound Steak Salad – Steak, lettuce, bleu cheese crumbles, red onions, red peppers, house vinaigrette, diced tomatoes, crispy onions, pretzel stick. Can substitute grilled chicken. I ask the waitperson to ask the chef to substitute grilled or sautéed onions for the crispy onions and to substitute extra diced tomatoes for the pretzel stick.

Napa Spinach Salad – Chicken, baby spinach, bacon, red onions, mushrooms, house vinaigrette, green apples, feta cheese, caramelized pecans, dried cranberries, and pretzel stick. I ask the waitperson to ask the chef to substitute extra mushrooms for the bacon and to substitute extra red onion for the pretzel stick.

Caesar Salad – Romaine lettuce, Caesar dressing, parmesan cheese, parmesan toasted croutons, pretzel stick. For an additional charge can add chicken breast. I ask the waitperson to ask the chef to substitute extra Romaine for the pretzel stick and to substitute bleu cheese dressing for the Caesar dressing.

Side Garden Salad

Side Caesar Salad – See Caesar Salad above.

Dressings: House vinaigrette, ranch, bleu cheese, honey mustard, fat free raspberry vinaigrette, or Italian.

Bowls:

Game Day Chili – Spicy chili, cheddar & Monterey Jack cheeses, sour cream, green onions, side of tortilla chips. I do not eat the tortilla chips.

Tomato Basil Soup – Served with pretzel stick. I do not eat the pretzel stick.

Sides:

Coleslaw

Broccoli

Street Tacos:

Three tacos served with chips and salsa. I do not eat the chips.

Chicken Tacos – Shredded seasoned chicken, cheddar & Monterey Jack cheeses, pico de gallo, grilled white corn tortilla.

 Steak Tacos – Shredded seasoned steak, cheddar & Monterey Jack cheeses, pico de gallo, grilled white corn tortilla.

Handhelds:

Hot Fox – Hand-battered chicken breast, classic buffalo sauce, lettuce,tomato, ranch or bleu cheese dressing on the side, served with fries. I ask the waitperson to ask the chef to leave off the batter and grill my chicken and to substitute a vegetable for the fries.

Black Forest – Grilled turkey, Bavarian pretzel roll, Applewood smoked bacon, Monterey jack cheese, lettuce, tomatoes, honey mustard, served with fries. I ask the waitperson to ask the chef to substitute extra turkey for the bacon and to substitute a vegetable for the fries.

Capri Panini – Chicken breast, Italian sourdough, spinach, Swiss cheese, tomatoes, basil pesto, sundried tomato mayonnaise, served with fries. I ask the waitperson to ask the chef to substitute a vegetable for the fries.

French Dip – London broil, ciabatta bun, au jus and horseradish on the side, served with fries. Cheese can be added for an additional charge. I ask the waitperson to ask the chef to substitute a vegetable for the fries.

All Star Burgers:

All burgers are served with fries. **S**ubstitute a veggie burger or chicken breast at no additional. On all burgers I ask the waitperson to ask the chef to substitute a vegetable for the fries.

Barnyard – Angus burger, Applewood smoked bacon, white American cheese, sunny-side up fried egg, mayonnaise on the side. I ask the waitperson to ask the chef to substitute cheddar cheese for the bacon and American cheese and to scramble the egg instead of frying it.

Stacked – Angus burger, Applewood smoked bacon, Swiss and bleu cheeses, caramelized onions, lettuce, tomato, red onions, and pickles. I ask the waitperson to ask the chef to substitute extra red onion for the bacon.

Classic Cheeseburger – Angus burger, lettuce, tomato, pickles, onions, choice of Swiss, cheddar, pepper Jack, American, provolone, or Monterey Jack cheese. I order any cheese except American.

<u>Ranch Hand</u> – Angus burger, pepper Jack cheese, Applewood smoked bacon, fried onion straws and ranch dressing. I ask the waitperson to ask the chef to substitute extra cheese for the bacon and to substitute grilled or sautéed onions for the fried onion straws.

<u>Mushroom Swiss</u> – Angus burger, sautéed mushrooms, Swiss cheese, lettuce, tomato, red onions, and pickles.

The Big Finish:

<u>The Great Cookie Blitz</u> – Chocolate chip cookie, vanilla ice cream and chocolate syrup.

<u>New York Style Cheesecake</u> – Strawberries, whipped cream, and strawberry purée.

Gas House Grill
Creve Coeur, MO

Appetizers:

Spinach Dip – Served with tortilla chips and loaf of buttered garlic bread. I ask the waitperson to ask the chef to leave off the buttered garlic bread.

Chili Cheese Nachos Supreme – Crispy corn tortilla chips topped with our famous chili, melted cheddar and Monterey Jack cheese, lettuce, tomatoes, black olives, and jalapenos. I ask the waitperson to ask the chef to leave off the jalapenos.

Sandwiches:

Served with your choice of fries, house made chips, coleslaw or cottage cheese. Substitute soup or a small salad for an additional charge. On all sandwiches I order the small salad.

Hall of Fame Buffalo Chicken Sandwich – Crispy deep fried large boneless breast of chicken, smothered in our buffalo sauce. With bleu cheese or ranch dressing sitting on the bench. I ask the waitperson to ask the chef to substitute grilled chicken for the deep fried chicken.

French Dip – Thinly sliced lean roast top round dipped in au jus, piled high on a toasted hoagie roll and a side of au jus. Add a melting of Swiss cheese and caramelized onions for an additional charge.

Slow Smoked Beef Brisket – A Gas House tradition! Thinly sliced mouthwatering slow smoked beef brisket, Jack Daniel's caramelized onions, BBQ sauce, and smoked aged cheddar cheese on grilled rosemary focaccia bread.

The Cuban – Grilled garlic and herb marinated chicken breast, smoked ham, banana peppers, spiced pickles, Swiss cheese, Cajun mayo on a ciabatta roll. I ask the waitperson to ask the chef to substitute tomatoes for the smoked ham.

Rueben – Warm thinly sliced corned beef, Bavarian sauerkraut, Thousand Island sauce, a melting of Swiss cheese on toasted marble rye. I ask the waitperson to ask the chef to substitute yellow mustard for the Thousand Island sauce.

Sam's Philly Cheese Steak – An authentic Philly cheesesteak sandwich! Lean roast sirloin, sautéed peppers, onions and a melting of Swiss cheese piled high on a toasted hoagie roll.

Cajun Chicken Philly – Cajun seasoned blackened chicken breast smothered in sautéed onions, peppers and a melting of Swiss cheese piled high on a toasted hoagie roll.

Smokehouse Chicken – Grilled marinated chicken breast, topped with grilled onions, hickory smoked bacon, BBQ sauce and melted cheddar cheese. I ask the waitperson to ask the chef to substitute extra grilled onions for the bacon.

Parmesan Chicken – Grilled marinated chicken breast, topped with our own marinara sauce, melted provolone cheese and served on a grilled rosemary focaccia roll.

Turkey Club – Sliced turkey breast, hickory smoked bacon, aged cheddar cheese, lettuce, tomato and mayo on seared sourdough bread. I ask the waitperson to ask the chef to substitute extra tomato for the bacon and to leave off the center slice of bread.

Salads:

House Salad – Mixed greens, tomato, cucumber, red onions, provel and dressing of your choice. I ask the waitperson to ask the chef to substitute extra tomato for the cucumber.

Buffalo Farmhand – Your choice of grilled or crispy fried chicken served buffalo style atop mixed greens. Gas House cheese blend, sweet red onion, bell peppers, cucumber and tomato. I order the grilled chicken and ask the waitperson to ask the chef to substitute extra sweet red onion for the cucumbers.

Grilled Chicken Caesar – Crisp romaine tossed with Romano cheese, seasoned croutons, diced tomatoes, Caesar dressing and topped with tender grilled chicken breast. I ask the waitperson to ask the chef to leave off the croutons and to substitute bleu cheese dressing for the Caesar dressing.

Anna's Italian Chop Salad – Chopped mixed greens, sweet red onion, tomato, black olives, bell pepper, banana peppers, mushrooms, pepperoni, ham, chicken, provel cheese and tossed in our sweet Italian dressing. I ask the waitperson to ask the chef to substitute extra chicken for the pepperoni and ham.

Pacific Coast – Broiled pacific cod atop mixed greens, toasted almonds, diced cranberry, feta cheese and dressed with fat free raspberry vinaigrette. A real customer favorite. I ask the waitperson to ask the chef to substitute chicken breast or turkey breast for the pacific cod.

California Coast – Mixed greens, toasted almonds, dried cranberry, feta cheese and dressed with fat free raspberry vinaigrette.

Spinach Salad – Baby spinach leaves, sweet red onion dried cranberry, fresh tomato, bacon, bleu cheese crumbles and dressed with balsamic vinaigrette. I ask the waitperson to ask the chef to substitute extra cranberry for the bacon.

Burgers:

Bison Burgers – It's back, bigger and better than ever!

All specialty burgers can be made with healthy alternative turkey burger with only 4 grams of fat. All burgers served with your choice of fries, house made chips, coleslaw or cottage cheese. Soup or salad can be substituted for an additional charge. I order the salad with my burger.

Bison Burger – A healthy alternative! A grilled juicy half pound bison burger.

Turkey Burger All white meat and delicious, another healthy alternative.

MVP Steak Burger – The classic! Grilled half pound sirloin burger. Add cheese for an additional charge.

Mushroom Swiss Burger – Grilled beef sirloin burger, three mustard herb glaze, sautéed mushrooms, crisp bacon and Swiss cheese. I ask the waitperson to ask the chef to substitute extra mushrooms for the bacon.

Bleu Moon Burger – Grilled beef sirloin burger on top of our Gas House onion straws, topped with baked creamy crumbled bleu cheese and A-1 sauce. I ask the waitperson to ask the chef to substitute grilled onions for the onion straws and to substitute mustard for the A-1 sauce.

Soups:

Bill's Chili

Baked French Onion Soup – I ask the waitperson to ask the chef to prepare my onion soup without any bread or croutons.

Entrees:

NY Strip – Grilled 8 oz. NY Strip grilled to perfection with garlic herbed butter served with baked potato and salad. I ask the waitperson to ask the chef to substitute a vegetable for the baked potato.

Nanette's Homemade Meatloaf – Our mom's secret recipe. A generous portion of meatloaf served with mashed potatoes and gravy, green beans and a piece of garlic toast. I ask the waitperson to ask the chef to substitute a small salad for the mashed potatoes and garlic toast.

Chicken Parmesan – Crisp fried chicken breast served over a bed of spaghetti with our homemade marinara and melted provel cheese. Served with a dinner salad and garlic toast. I ask the waitperson to ask the chef to substitute grilled chicken for the crispy fried chicken and to leave off the garlic toast.

Baked Cannelloni – Tubular noodles stuffed with seasoned Italian beef, topped with our homemade marinara and melted provel cheese. Served with a dinner salad and garlic toast. I ask the waitperson to ask the chef to leave off the garlic toast.

Gas House Grill's Specialty:

Stone oven pizza – All pizzas are 12" and St. Louis style thin crust.

Fresh Veggie Pizza – Topped with fresh tomatoes, red onions, black olives, peppers, mushrooms and spinach.

Sweet Baby Ray's BBQ Chicken Pizza – Sweet Baby Ray's BBQ sauce, grilled chicken, bacon, red onion and provel chicken. I ask the waitperson to ask the chef to substitute mushrooms for the bacon.

Buffalo Chicken – Grilled chicken, sweet red onion, crisp bacon, our very own wing sauce, and provel cheese drizzled with ranch dressing. I ask the waitperson to ask the chef to substitute bell peppers for the crisp bacon.

Build Your Own – Cheese pizza. Additional toppings available for an extra charge.

Hamburger

Grilled Chicken

Bell Peppers

Mushrooms

Black Olives

Banana Peppers

Spinach

Sweet Red Onion

O'Niell's
Albuquerque, NM

Starters:

Crispy Corned Beef & Cabbage Egg Rolls

Soups:

Bowl or Cup

Lamb Stew

Salads:

Add a char-broiled chicken breast to any salad for an additional charge.

Fresh Spinach Salad

Bleu Cheese & Sirloin Salad

O'Niell's Fabulous Caesar Salad – Romaine lettuce, parmesan cheese, fresh croutons and our house made dressing. I ask the waitperson to ask the waiter to substitute bleu cheese dressing for the Caesar dressing and to leave off the croutons.

Celtic Favorites:

Shepherd's Pie

Bangers & Mash – I ask the waitperson to ask the chef to substitute a vegetable for the mash potatoes.

Steak, Fish & Chicken:

Sirloin & Boxty – I ask the waitperson to ask the chef to substitute a vegetable for the boxty.

Marinated Chicken Kabob – I ask the waitperson to ask the chef to substitute a vegetable for the rice pilaf.

Smothered Chicken Breast – I ask the waitperson to ask the chef to substitute a vegetable for the rice and potato.

Burgers:

All of our burgers, sandwiches and Ruebens are served with your choice of coleslaw, side salad, fruit or a cup of soup.

O'Niell's Black & Bleu Burger

BYOB – Build your own burger or garden burger or Portobello burger. Served with lettuce, tomato and onion. Choose from the following toppings: Swiss, Monterey Jack, provolone, Cheddar or Bleu chesses: green chile, mushrooms or grilled onions for an additional charge.

Garden Burger in Paradise

O'Niell's Burger in Paradise – Award winning! Seasoned ground beef broiled to order and served with lettuce, onion, tomato, American cheese, bacon and green chile on a Kaiser roll. I ask the waitperson to ask the chef to substitute cheddar cheese for the American cheese and to substitute extra tomato for the bacon.

Ruebens:

Choose your side from the choices listed under burgers.

Rob's Rueben – Grilled corned beef, sauerkraut, Russian dressing and Swiss cheese on light rye bread. Make it veggie! Substitute a seasoned Portobello mushroom. I ask the waitperson to ask the chef to substitute spicy mustard for the Russian dressing.

Boxty Rueben – I ask the waitperson to ask the chef to substitute spicy mustard for the Russian dressing.

Apple Rueben – Grilled, sweet-tart apple slices for the corned beef in a classic Rueben. I ask the waitperson to ask the chef to substitute raspberry vinaigrette for the Russian dressing.

Sandwiches:

Choose your side from the choices listed under burgers.

St. Patty Melt – Ground beef seasoned just like the burger, cooked medium, on grilled rye bread with Swiss cheese and sautéed onions. Make it a veggie-sub Portobello mushroom.

Grilled Philly Sandwich

Steak Sandwich

Southwest French Dip

Buffalo Chicken Sandwich – The heat of our award-winning wing sauce is balanced perfectly by the freshness of ripe red tomatoes, lettuce, and onion. Add bleu cheese dressing for a classic combo.

Char-Broiled Chicken Breast – Monterey style or Cajun style.

Turkey Jack – Grilled sliced turkey breast, Jack cheese, and green chile on fresh sourdough.

Desserts:

The Chocolate Celebration

Chocolate Decadence

Patrick's Restaurant & Sports Bar
Maryland Heights, MO

Lunch Specials:

Lunch Soup and Salad – Chef's daily seasonal soup, French onion soup or Chili and a House side salad or Caesar side salad. If I order the Caesar side salad, I ask the waitperson to ask the chef to substitute bleu cheese dressing for the Caesar dressing and to leave off the croutons.

Half Sandwich and Soup or Salad – One half of our Mesquite Breast Turkey and either an appetizer portion of our House or Caesar Salad or a cup or our white bean or chef's daily soup.

Luncheon Salads – Select a lunch sized portion of our regular selection of salads. Choose from an Asian Chicken, Cobb Salad, Albert's Wedge Salad or Classic Chicken Caesar Salad. If I order the Classic Chicken Caesar Salad, I ask the waitperson to ask the chef to substitute bleu cheese dressing for the Caesar dressing and to leave off the croutons.

Luncheon Favorites:

Lunch Sized Portion of our Homemade Meatloaf.

Arroz con Pollo – Lunch sized portion of Albert's Favorite Dominican Chicken and rice dish. I ask the waitperson to ask the chef to substitute a vegetable for the rice.

Charbroiled Breast of Chicken – With Yukon whipped potato and chef's daily vegetable. I ask the waitperson to ask the chef to substitute extra vegetables for the whipped potatoes.

Appetizers:

Spinach Dip – Spinach, three cheeses and roasted artichoke dip with crispy corn tortillas.

Buffalo Chicken Strips – Traditional style with Wasabi Honey

Mustard. Buffalo style tossed in tangy Pujol's Buffalo Sauce. I ask the waitperson to ask the chef to substitute grilled chicken for the fried chicken.

Angus Sliders – Three bite size Angus burgers served on our mini brioche buns with caramelized onions, lettuce, tomato, dill pickle chips and Chipotle sauce.

Mini Burger Blue Sliders – Three mini Angus beef sliders, charbroiled and served with Hickory Smoked Bacon, blue cheese, lettuce, vine ripe tomato and a splash of our signature Bourbon barbecue sauce on a soft brioche bun. I ask the waitperson to ask the chef to substitute extra tomato for the bacon.

Fajita Steak Quesadilla – Sirloin steak topped with onions peppers, pico de gallo and cheese rolled in a flour tortilla and served with fire roasted salsa.

French Onion Soup – I ask the waitperson to ask the chef to prepare my soup without bread or croutons.

Chef's Daily Seasonal Soup

Salads:

Wedge Salad – Wedge of iceberg lettuce, bacon, tomatoes, chopped egg and your choice of house made dressings. I ask the waitperson to ask the chef to substitute extra tomato for the bacon.

Julian's House Salad – Add chicken for an extra charge. A blend of baby greens, iceberg and romaine lettuce, tomato, red onion, olives, cucumber, carrot and hard cooked egg with your choice of house made dressing. I ask the waitperson to ask the chef to substitute extra carrot for the cucumber.

Chop House Cobb Salad – Herb marinated and grilled breast of chicken, crisp greens, tomato, avocado, blue cheese, red and green onion, Hickory Smoked Bacon and hard cooked egg all tossed in your choice of our house made dressing. I ask the waitperson to ask the chef to substitute extra red and green onion for the bacon.

<u>Asian Chicken Salad</u> – Hoisin marinated breast of chicken, Napa cabbage, green onions, red bell pepper shredded carrot, bamboo shoots and water chestnuts all tossed in our spicy cilantro peanut dressing.

<u>Caesar Salad</u> – Charbroiled breast of chicken with crispy romaine, parmesan cheese, and house made croutons and a creamy Caesar dressing. I ask the waitperson to ask the chef to substitute blue cheese dressing for the Caesar dressing and to leave off the croutons.

<u>Steak Salad</u> – Southwestern marinated and charbroiled flat iron steak, crispy iceberg lettuce, fire roasted red peppers, roasted corn salsa, crumbled blue cheese, red and green onions all tossed in our smoked jalapeno buttermilk dressing. I ask the waitperson to ask the chef to substitute blue cheese dressing for the smoked jalapeno buttermilk dressing.

<u>Hall of Fame Salad</u> – Grilled chicken blue cheese, haricot verts, strawberries, grapes and spicy pecans in our house made dressing. I ask the waitperson to ask the chef to substitute extra strawberries for the grapes.

Burgers:

All of our burgers are served with lettuce, vine ripened tomato & a pickle. All burgers & sandwiches are served with seasoned French fries. On all burgers and sandwiches I ask the waitperson to ask the chef to substitute a vegetable for the fries.

<u>Angus Burger</u> – Angus beef half pound chuck burger, charbroiled and served with lettuce, vine ripe tomato and on a soft brioche bun. Cheese can be added for an additional charge.

Bison Burger – One third pound of lean ground buffalo charbroiled to order. Served on a brioche bun with lettuce and tomato. I order it with the coleslaw.

Grilled Turkey Burger – Combined with fresh garlic and spices. Served on a brioche bun with lettuce and tomato. I order it with the coleslaw.

Mushroom Burger – Angus beef half pound chuck burger, charbroiled and served with sauté of mushrooms and caramelized onion, Swiss cheese, lettuce and vine ripe tomato on a soft brioche bun.

Burger Blue – Angus beef pound chuck burger, charbroiled and served with Hickory Smoked Bacon, crumbled blue cheese, lettuce, vine ripe tomato and a splash of our signature Bourbon barbecue sauce on a soft brioche bun. I ask the waitperson to ask the chef to substitute red onion for the bacon.

Steaks:

12 oz. Grilled Ribeye Steak – Thick cut and served with steak butter and chef's seasonal vegetables.

12 oz. New York Strip Steak – Thick cut and dry aged strip steak served with steak butter and chef's seasonal vegetables.

8 oz. Filet – Dry aged filet served with Yukon Gold Whipped Potatoes, mushrooms, a red wine reduction and chef's seasonal vegetables. I ask the waitperson to ask the chef to substitute extra seasonal vegetables for the whipped potatoes.

Sandwiches:

All sandwiches are served with seasoned French fries. On all sandwiches I ask the waitperson to ask the chef to substitute a vegetable for the fries.

Chicken Ciabatta BLT – Char-Grilled Chicken breast melted Provolone Cheese, Applewood Smoked Bacon, basil pesto mayonnaise, lettuce & tomato on ciabatta bread. I ask the waitperson to ask the chef to substitute extra tomato for the bacon.

Turkey Sandwich – Mesquite smoked turkey, thinly sliced and served with Provolone Cheese, lettuce, tomato, onion and creamy mayonnaise on soft wheat bread.

Roast Beef – Oven roasted and thinly sliced with caramelized sweet onion, melted Provolone Cheese, fried onion straws on toasted Italian bun with French onion jus. I ask the waitperson to ask the chef to substitute grilled onion for the fried onion straws.

Corned Beef Reuben – Shaved corned beef piled high with sauerkraut, melted Swiss cheese and smoked tomato aioli on toasted New York style rye bread.

Prime Rib Sandwich – 7 oz. cut of prime rib, grilled and topped with onions, peppers & Provel cheese. I ask the waitperson to ask the chef to substitute Swiss cheese for the Provel cheese.

Chicken Salad Sandwich – House made with almonds, lettuce, tomato and red onion. Served on a croissant with coleslaw.

Grilled Portabella Sandwich – A giant portabella mushroom marinated in balsamic vinegar with herbs, served on a brioche bun with lettuce, tomato, grilled red onions, melted Provel cheese and spicy chipotle dressing. Served with coleslaw. I ask the waitperson to ask the chef to substitute Swiss cheese for the Provel cheese.

Pizza:

Margherita Pizza – Fresh tomato, basil & mozzarella.

Mozzarella Pizza – Roasted tomato, fresh spinach, artichoke & garlic.

Mediterranean Pizza – Fire roasted red pepper sauce with fresh spinach, grilled chicken, feta cheese and Kalamata olives.

BBQ Chicken Pizza – Roasted chicken breast, BBQ sauce, vine ripe tomato, onion, fresh cilantro topped with mozzarella and provolone cheese.

Buffalo Chicken – Grilled chicken in buffalo sauce & onions.

Bacon Cheeseburger – Hamburger, bacon, onion with cheddar, provel & mozzarella cheese with a tangy mustard ketchup sauce. I ask the waitperson to ask the chef to substitute Swiss cheese for the provel and to substitute extra onion for the bacon.

Entrees:

Served with House Salad, Caesar Salad or Soup of the Day.

Greek Chicken Breast – 12 oz. bone-in-breast of chicken served Greek style with virgin olive oil, fresh lemon, Kalamata olives, oregano and garlic over whipped potato and roasted seasonal vegetables with a jus. We will finish the dish with feta cheese. I ask the waitperson to ask the chef to substitute extra seasonal vegetables for the whipped potato.

Herb Roasted Chicken Breast – 12 oz. bone-in breast of chicken served over whipped Yukon gold potato and roasted seasonal vegetables with natural pan jus. I ask the waitperson to ask the chef to substitute extra seasonal vegetables for the Yukon gold potato.

Mile High Meatloaf – Combined with ground chuck, onions, tomato, and celery. Served with fried onion straws and roasted garlic whipped Yukon gold potato. I ask the waitperson to ask the chef to substitute grilled onions for the fried onion straws and to substitute seasonal vegetables for the Yukon gold potato.

Fettuccini Pasta – Fettuccini tossed with vine ripe tomato, roasted garlic, mushrooms, basil and cream topped with grilled chicken, parmesan and pine nuts.

Pasta Fresca Penne – Penne noodles served with sundried tomatoes, broccoli, garlic, peppers, spinach and tossed in extra virgin olive oil and parmesan cheese. Can add chicken for an additional charge.

Sides:

Poppyseed Coleslaw

Cup of Seasonal Fruit

Seasonal Vegetables

Decadent, Delicious Desserts:

Try one of our fantastic house made desserts. Your taste buds will love you.

Carrot Cake – Sweet, moist spice cake, full of carrots and toasted walnuts than covered with thick layers of gooey pecan crème cheese icing!

Serious Chocolate Brownie – Decadent and rich, chocolate brownie with a hint of vanilla, served with Tahitian vanilla ice crème, a chocolate lovers dream!

Crème Brulee – A rich, silky vanilla bean custard topped with caramelized sugar, need we say more...fantastic!

Rustic Apple Tart – A free form apple tart with flaky crust, seasoned just right and served warm with premium vanilla ice cream, just what you wanted.

Satchmo's Bar & Grill
Chesterfield, MO

Greens and Wraps:

Dressing: Honey Mustard, French, Italian, Greek Feta Vinaigrette, and Bleu Cheese.

House Salad – Fresh greens, tomato wedge, chopped bacon, cucumbers, egg & red onions. I ask the waitperson to ask the chef to substitute extra greens for the chopped bacon and the cucumbers.

Chef Salad – Fresh lettuce topped with diced ham, turkey Jack & cheddar cheese, tomato & bacon. I ask the waitperson to ask the chef to substitute extra turkey for the ham and to substitute extra tomato for the bacon.

Grilled Chicken Salad – Grilled chicken, tomato, sliced egg, cucumber, onion & chopped bacon. I ask the waitperson to ask the chef to substitute extra tomato for the cucumber and the chopped bacon.

Chris' Chopped Steakhouse Salad – Fresh greens, cucumber, tomatoes, bacon, black olives, red peppers & onions with gorgonzola. Tossed in our creamy garlic feta dressing & topped with grilled steak. I ask the waitperson to ask the chef to substitute extra tomatoes for the cucumber and the bacon.

Chopped Salad – Fresh greens, cucumber, tomatoes, bacon, black olives, red peppers and onions with gorgonzola. Tosseds in our creamy garlic feta dressing. I ask the waitperson to ask the chef to substitute extra fresh greens for the cucumber and to substitute extra red peppers for the bacon.

Caesar Salad – Traditional Caesar Salad. Grilled chicken can be added for an additional charge. I order it with the grilled chicken. I ask the waitperson to ask the chef to substitute bleu cheese dressing for the Caesar dressing and to leave off the croutons.

Cobb Salad – Fresh lettuce with tomato, sliced egg, cucumber, bleu cheese, turkey & bacon. I ask the waitperson to ask the chef to substitute extra lettuce for the cucumber and to substitute extra turkey for the bacon.

Baja Explosion – Fajita grilled chicken, mixed cheese, corn relish, cilantro, diced tomato, crispy tortilla strips with our avocado ranch dressing. Served with grilled cheese quesadilla wedges topped with a bit of our Green Chili Verde. I ask the waitperson to ask the chef to substitute extra tomato for the tortilla strips and to substitute bleu cheese dressing for the avocado ranch dressing.

The Greek – A rough country salad of juicy tomatoes, crisp cucumber, sliced red onion, green pepper, pepperoncini, crumbly feta cheese and plump Kalamata olives with our Greek Feta Vinaigrette. I ask the waitperson to ask the chef to substitute extra green peppers for the cucumber.

Buffalo Chicken Wrap – Spicy breaded chicken tossed in Satchmo's wing sauce, romaine lettuce, provel cheese, avocado ranch dressing, chopped tomatoes and chives in a whole wheat tortilla with sweet potato fries. I ask the waitperson to ask the chef to substitute grilled chicken for the breaded chicken, to substitute bleu cheese dressing for the avocado ranch dressing, and to substitute a vegetable for the sweet potato fries.

Mediterranean Veggie Wrap – Garlic hummus, grilled red bell peppers, fresh romaine, fire roasted tomatoes, feta, cucumbers, red onion, zesty cherry peppers & cracked red pepper aioli, flour tortilla & sweet potato fries. I ask the waitperson to ask the chef to substitute a vegetable for the sweet potato fries.

The Cups & Bowls:

Soup & House Salad

Soup of the Day

Satchmo's Chili

Tavern Fare:

Eclectic American Bar Food.

Chesterfield Philly – Roast beef with Swiss cheese, green peppers & grilled onions served on a hoagie roll.

Smokehouse Grilled Chicken – Grilled chicken breast, cheddar cheese, Satchmo's own BBQ sauce & crisp bacon topped with an onion ring. I ask the waitperson to ask the chef to substitute lettuce for the bacon and the onion ring.

The Brick – Seasoned roast beef with Jack cheese, served on thick Texas toast with au jus.

Turkey Melt – Hand shaved smoked turkey with Jack cheese, tomato & bacon all melted on Texas toast. I ask the waitperson to ask the chef to substitute extra tomato for the bacon.

Burgers:

Smokehouse Burger – Topped with bacon, Cheddar, BBQ sauce & an onion ring. I ask the waitperson to ask the chef to substitute lettuce for the bacon and onion ring.

Cheeseburger – Your choice of American, Cheddar, Jack, Swiss, Provel, pepper of bleu cheese. I order any cheese except American.

Justa Burger – Just a plain ole burger, but delicious none-the-less.

Satchmo's Southwest Burger – Southwest Chipotle sauce, Jack cheese, grilled jalapenos & red onions. I ask the waitperson to ask the chef to substitute grilled tomato for the grilled jalapenos.

Bison Burger – Lean bison beef, grilled & topped to your liking.

Southwest Fare:

Chris' travel often takes him into the Southwestern US and Texas – he loves the fresh flavors, grilled meats, salsa & sauces – enjoy that influence in our new Southwestern Fare section.

Quesadilla's – Your choice of cheese, chicken, or beef with green onions, cheese, tomatoes & our fresh salsa.

Tequila Chicken Sandwich – Marinated in tequila lime sauce, grilled & topped with jalapenos. Santa Fe slaw, pepper cheese & our homemade verde sauce. I ask the waitperson to ask the chef to substitute tomatoes for the jalapenos.

Satchmo's Signature Items:

All sandwiches & burgers are served with a pickle spear & your choice of coleslaw or cottage cheese.

Bre's Italian Sandwich – Roast beef, ham, salami, Swiss cheese, lettuce, pepperoncini, tomatoes, red onions & our house sauce served on a warm hoagie roll. I ask the waitperson to ask the chef to substitute extra roast beef for the ham.

Chris' Steak Sandwich – Dry rubbed NY Strip cooked to a light pink center, served on a toasted hoagie roll with Chris' secret mayo. Topped with grilled onions & sautéed cherry peppers. Add cheese for an additional charge. Chris recommends feta.

Tuscan Pesto Chicken – Pesto chicken breast, mozzarella cheese, sliced tomato, shredded romaine & sun-dried tomato spread with a small Greek salad.

Pizza:

The Cheeser Pizza – Extra, extra cheese.

The Margherita – Diced tomatoes, chopped garlic, mozzarella & parmesan cheese with fresh basil and drizzle of olive oil.

Pat's BBQ Chicken Pizza – Satchmo's BBQ sauce with

cheese, breaded chicken chunks & red onion. I ask the waitperson to ask the chef to substitute grilled chicken for the breaded chicken.

Build Your Own – We got all kinds of stuff back in the kitchen. So build your own.

Toppings:

Chicken

Hamburger

Artichokes

Green Peppers

Red Peppers

White Onion

Red Onion

Mushrooms

Hot Sauces

Tomato Sauce

Pesto Sauce

BBQ Sauce

Spinach

Pepperoncini

Olives

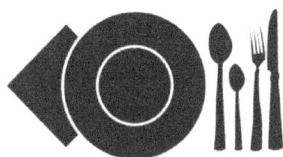

BUFFETS

Bonanza Steakhouse
International Chain Restaurant

All You Can Eat Buffet – Salads, vegetables, pasta and desserts.

½ Pound Sirloin – USDA Choice.

10 oz. Top Sirloin – Center cut.

10 oz. Ribeye

1 lb. T-Bone

Sirloin Tips

Chicken Monterey or Grilled Chicken

Three Steak Medallions

Chopped Steak

½ Pound Cheeseburger or Grilled Chicken Sandwich

Senior Lunch Buffet

Senior Dinner Buffet

Golden Corral
Chain Restaurant – All you can eat buffet

<u>Everyday Menu Items:</u>

<u>Assorted Steamed Vegetables</u>

<u>Awesome Pot Roast</u>

<u>Bourbon Street Chicken</u>

<u>Broccoli</u>

<u>Cabbage</u>

<u>Carrot Cake</u>

<u>Carrots</u>

<u>Cauliflower</u>

<u>Chocolate Cake w/ Chocolate Frosting</u>

<u>Coleslaw</u>

<u>Fresh Fruit</u>

<u>Fudgy Brownies</u>

<u>Green Beans</u>

<u>Pasta</u>

<u>Cheese Pizza</u>

<u>Greens</u>

<u>Grilled-to-order USDA Sirloin Steaks (*dinner only)</u>

<u>Meatloaf</u>

<u>Rotisserie Chicken</u>

<u>50+ Toppings on our Fresh Cold Salad Bar</u>

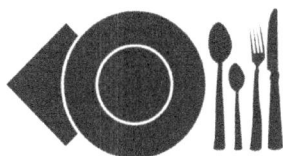

COMEDY CLUBS

Cold Water Fusion Restaurant & Comedy Club
Albuquerque, NM

Appetizers:

Spinach & Artichoke Dip – Served with toasted French bread.

Soups & Salads:

Served for brunch, lunch and dinner.

Soup of the Day

Spinach Salad – Fresh organic spinach with bell & sweet peppers, tomatoes, sunflower seeds, feta cheese and red wine vinaigrette. Can add chicken for an additional charge.

Side Spring Mix Salad – Organic mixed greens including radicchio oak leaf lettuce and endive served with Kalamata olives, sunflower seeds, feta cheese with our red wine vinaigrette.

Full Wedge Salad – Quartered iceberg lettuce with bacon and shaved carrots, with your choice of dressing: blue cheese dressing with blue cheese crumbles, house vinaigrette and feta cheese, red wine vinaigrette and feta cheese, or ranch with cheddar cheese. I ask the waitperson to ask the chef to leave off the bacon.

Dinner Entre Selections:

Sirloin Steak- 10 ounce hand cut and char-grilled garnished with pickled onion and Chimichurri sauce. Served with the vegetable and starch of the day.

Boneless Short Ribs – Braised beef with red wine and chilies and plums slow cooked with celery, onions and carrots. Served with the vegetable and starch of the day.

Turkey Osso Bucco – Braised turkey on the bone with white wine and roasted celery, onions, and carrots. Served with the vegetable and starch of the day.

Mediterranean Fettuccini al Pesto – Pesto fettuccini with tomatoes diced Kalamata olives and diced artichoke hearts. Chicken can be added for an additional charge.

Coldwater Burger – ½ pound hamburger with red chile glazed bacon, roasted green chile and pepper Jack cheese. Served with house made potato chips. I ask the waitperson to ask the chef to substitute tomato for the red chile glazed bacon and to substitute a vegetable for the potato chips.

Lunch Menu:

Lunch Entrée Sandwiches, Tacos, and New Mexican Favorites Ala Carte.

Coldwater Burger – ½ pound hamburger with red chile glazed bacon, roasted green chile and pepper Jack cheese served on a handmade bun with aioli and grain mustard. Lettuce, tomato and pickles served upon request. I ask the waitperson to ask the chef to substitute tomato for the red chile glazed bacon.

Cajun Chicken Sandwich – Blackened chicken, pepper Jack cheese, sautéed sweet peppers, aioli and grain mustard on a black poppy seed bun.

Honey Mustard Chicken Sandwich – Homemade honey mustard glaze grilled chicken, red chile glazed bacon, Swiss cheese melted on a black poppy seed bun. I ask the waitperson to ask the chef to substitute tomato for the red chile glazed bacon.

Hamburger – ½ pound burger on a handmade bun with aioli and grain mustard. Lettuce, tomato and pickles served upon request.

Add any side of your choice:

Sautéed Green Beans

Spring Mix Salad – Available for an additional charge.

World Specialty Lunch Entrée Combinations:

Quiche of the Day/France – Served with ½ spring mix salad. Organic mixed greens including radicchio oak leaf lettuce and endive served with Kalamata olives, sunflower seeds and feta cheese with our red wine vinaigrette.

Tuscan Turkey Wrap/Italy – Turkey salad with bacon, feta cheese, lettuce, cucumber slices wrapped in a spinach tortilla. Served with a ½ spring mix salad. Organic mixed greens including radicchio oak leaf lettuce and endive served with Kalamata olives, sunflower seeds and feta cheese with our red wine vinaigrette. I ask the waitperson to ask the chef to substitute tomatoes for the bacon and cucumbers.

Gluten Free Lunch Options:

Cajun Chicken Combo – Blackened chicken, pepper Jack cheese, sautéed sweet peppers, served with spring mix salad. Organic mixed greens including radicchio oak leaf lettuce and endive served with Kalamata olives, sunflower seeds and feta cheese with our red wine vinaigrette.

Honey Mustard Chicken Combo – 8 oz. honey mustard glaze chicken breast, red chile glazed bacon, and melted Swiss cheese. Served with a spring mix salad. Organic mixed greens including radicchio oak leaf lettuce and endive served with Kalamata olives, sunflower seeds and feta cheese with our red wine vinaigrette. I ask the waitperson to ask the chef to substitute tomatoes for the bacon.

Breakfast Selections:

Spinach & Artichoke Dip – Served with toasted French bread.

Steak and Eggs – 6 ounce sirloin steak with two eggs and seasoned potatoes. I ask the waitperson to ask the chef to substitute sliced tomatoes for the potatoes.

Crepes of the Day – Your choice of "sweet" or "savory" crepes of the day. Served with seasoned potatoes. I ask the waitperson to ask the chef to substitute spring mix salad for the potatoes.

Four Course Meal for (2):

First Course/Soup or Traditional Caesar Salad – If I order the salad, I ask the waitperson to have the chef substitute blue cheese dressing for the Caesar dressing.

Second Course/Spinach and Artichoke Dip – With toasted French bread.

Main Course/Choice Of:

Grilled Flat Iron Steak – Garnished with pickled onion and Chimichurri sauce. Served with garlic mashed potatoes and sautéed green beans. I ask the waitperson to ask the chef to substitute a spring mix salad for the potatoes.

Blackened Chicken – (gluten free) with grilled sweet peppers and melted pepperjack cheese. Served with dirty rice and sautéed green beans. I ask the waitperson to ask the chef to substitute a spring mix salad for the dirty rice.

Spinach and Mozzarella Raviolis – (vegetarian) served with housemade marinara sauce and parmesan cheese.

Dessert/Choice of:

Crème Brulee – Vanilla or fruit flavored.

Bread Pudding – A house favorite served with caramel sauce and ice cream.

Brownie Bottom Pie – (gluten free) with ice cream and chocolate sauce.

Desserts:

Bread Pudding – Ala mode with ice cream. Our non-traditional spin on bread pudding with no raisins or nuts.

Crème Brulee of the Day

Dessert Du Jour – Ask your server for the featured dessert of the day.

INTERNATIONAL CHAIN RESTAURANTS

FROM FAT TO FABULOUS™:
Applebee's
Denny's
Longhorn Steakhouse
Panera Bread Co/St. Louis Bread Co.
T.G.I.Fridays

WE WENT FROM FAT TO FABULOUS™
Maggiano's Little Italy
Olive Garden
Panera/St. Louis Bread Co.
Marriott Hotel Chain

THEY WENT FROM FAT TO FABULOUS TOGETHER™
Bonanza Steak House
Chili's
Corner Bakery
KFC
McDonalds
Outback Steakhouse
Ponderosa Steakhouse
Rainforest Café
Red Robin
Ruby Tuesday
Steak n' Shake
Tony Roma's

US CHAIN RESTAURANTS

FROM FAT TO FABULOUS™
Canyon Café/Sam's Café
Cheesecake Factory

First Watch
Granite City Food & Brewery
IHOP International
La Madeleine
P.F. Chang

WE WENT FROM FAT TO FABULOUS™

Black Angus Steakhouse
Boston Market
Bravo!/Brio
Buffalo Wild Wings Grill & Bar
California Pastrami
Canyon Café/ Sam's Café – Southwestern Grill
Carrabba's Italian Grill
Cheeseburger Cheeseburger
Colton's Steak House & Grill
Dion's
First Watch
Five Guys® Burgers & Fries
Five Star Burgers
Flying Star
Fuddruckers
Grand Traverse Pie Co.
HuHot Mongolian Grill
Jason's Deli
Logan's Roadhouse
McAllister's Deli
Mimi's Café
Montana Mike's Steakhouse
Newk's® Express Cafe
O'Charley's
Rafferty's Restaurant & Bar
Rib Crib
Romano's Macaroni Grill
Ruth's Chris Steak House

Saltgrass Steak House
Tahoe Joe's
Texas Roadhouse
Whole Hog Cafe
Ya Ya's – Euro Bistro
Zea Rotisserie Grill
Zio's Italian Kitchen

SUPERMARKET CHAINS:

Albertsons
Dierberg's Kitchens
Smith's/Kroger's
Sprouts Farmers Market – Country Kitchen
Whole Foods Market – Catering Menu

THEY WENT FROM FAT TO FABULOUS TOGETHER™

Bandanas
Basil's Kitchen & Bar/Hilton
Claim Jumper
Cooper's Hawk Winery & Restaurant
Dickey's Barbecue Pit
Elephant Bar
Firehouse Subs
Fox & Hound
Golden Corral
Houlihan's
La Salsa
Mimi's Café
Noodles & Company
The Old Spaghetti Factory
Tucanos Brazilian Grill
Whataburger

Visit Red Carpet Press
online at
www.Red-Carpet-Press.com

Keep up on our latest new
releases from your favorite
authors, as well as author
appearances, news, blogs,
chats, special offers and
more.

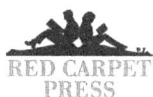

RED CARPET
PRESS

"Rolling Out the 'Read' Carpet, One Fantastic Book at a Time.™"

THE AUTHOR, E. S. ABRAMSON

ELAINE ABRAMSON, WRITING AS E. S. ABRAMSON, is an award-winning artist and author. She is a Pulitzer and Nobel Prize nominee, the first woman State Artist of Texas, and a Cleveland Heights High School hall of famer. Her artwork and writing have been on TV, the Internet, the radio, in major newspapers, used in Texas tourism, and on licensed merchandise.

She worked with Viacom Entertainment and the Pixelon Network, and is a former director of the Animagic International Animation Studio School.

Ms. Abramson, her husband, and their Labrador retriever live in St. Louis and Albuquerque.

Visit the author's website at www.ElaineAbramson.com.

All editions of *FROM FAT TO FABULOUS: A DIET GUIDE FOR RESTAURANT LOVERS*™ are available in eBook and paperback format online and in book stores. Ask your favorite bookseller to order them for you.

HAPPY EATING,

ELAINE

www.ingramcontent.com/pod-product-compliance
Lightning Source LLC
Chambersburg PA
CBHW031147270326
41931CB00006B/176